I0896494

THE TAO OF ADDICTION *and* RECOVERY

"In this book, you will discover easy-to-follow Chi Kung practices to aid your recovery, as the authors systematically explain the nature and development of addictions, the process of recovery, and how the *Tao Te Ching* can provide guidance. In this book the authors also show readers how to heal sick and stuck emotions by addressing the urges and attitudes that often cause relapse."

William U. Wei, coauthor of *Living in the Tao* and *Sexual Reflexology*

THE TAO OF ADDICTION *and* RECOVERY

Chi Kung Practices for Restoring the Energy Flow in Mind and Body

MANTAK CHIA
AND
DOUG HILTON

DESTINY BOOKS

Destiny Books
Rochester, Vermont

Destiny Books
One Park Street
Rochester, Vermont 05767
www.DestinyBooks.com

Destiny Books is a division of Inner Traditions International

Originally published in Thailand in 2023 by Universal Healing Tao Publications under the title *The Tao of Addiction and Recovery: Discover the Way of Tao to be Clean, Sober, Healthy and Happy.*

Cataloging-in-Publication Data for this title is available from the Library of Congress

ISBN 979-8-88850-281-5 (print)
ISBN 979-8-88850-282-2 (ebook)

Printed and bound in India by Replika Press Pvt. Ltd.

10 9 8 7 6 5 4 3 2 1

Text design and layout by K. Manseau
This book was typeset in Garamond Premier Pro with Present LT Std and Sho LT Std used as display typefaces.

To send correspondence to the author of this book, mail a first-class letter to the author c/o Inner Traditions, One Park Street, Rochester, VT 05767, and we will forward the communication.

Contents

Acknowledgments

The authors and Universal Healing Tao Publications staff involved in the preparation and production of this book extend our gratitude to the many generations of Taoist masters who have passed on the knowledge of their lineage in the form of an unbroken oral transmission over thousands of years. In particular we thank Taoist Master Yi Eng (One Cloud Hermit) for his openness in transmitting the formulas of Taoist Inner Alchemy.

We offer our eternal gratitude to our parents and teachers for their many gifts to us, which have been crucial to our presentation of the Universal Healing Tao. Remembering them brings joy and satisfaction to our ongoing work.

We wish to thank the thousands of unknown men and women of the Taoist healing arts who developed many of the methods and ideas presented in this book. We also wish to thank our fellow Taoists, students, clients, families, and friends who have inspired the writing of this book by encouraging us to shed light on this important subject and to communicate the principles of Taoist Emotional Recycling to a wider audience.

The authors would like to express gratitude for the patience, thoroughness, and creativity that Colin Drown brought to the editing process for the first edition of this book.

Doug Hilton would like to thank the following individuals: first and foremost, Master Mantak Chia, for all of his knowledge, wisdom, guidance, and support; Dell Graff, for introducing him to the field of addictions counseling; Veronica Graff, for introducing him to the value of older traditions; Brent Neumann, for numerous thought-provoking conversations; Donna Baird, for introducing him to Eye Movement Desensitization and Reprocessing (EMDR) and for her continual support; Dr. Sal Mendaglio, for introducing him to the concept of polarities; Gerald Hilton, for his encouragement and continual reminders of the value of polar opposites; Edward Gutierrez, for his wisdom and constant encouragement; Jutta and Walter Kellenberger, for their quiet and steady support; Gordon Mah, for offering a patient and encouraging ear; Dr. Marshall Wilensky, for teaching EMDR to him; Dr. Francine Shapiro, for discovering EMDR; Dr. Robert Miller, for creating the Feeling State Addiction Protocol; and all the countless Taoist masters who contributed to the current knowledge.

Doug would also like to acknowledge that the opportunity for the ancient ways, teachings, and wisdom of Taoism to now be applied to modern-day problems would not have been possible without the tireless efforts of Master Chia to introduce the Universal Healing Tao system to the West.

Doug offers thanks to his wife, Ana, for her steady encouragement to share the value of the Taoist practices with the world. His brother, Gerry, must also be thanked for continually showing him that opposite ways are not necessarily bad, and this has helped Doug to move away from dualistic reality. Doug extends special thanks to William U. Wei, the Tao Garden production staff, and the editorial staff at Inner Traditions for their guidance and patience in helping to make this book a reality.

Putting The Tao of Addiction and Recovery into Practice

The information presented in this book is based on the authors' personal experience with and knowledge of the Tao of addiction and recovery. The practices described here have been used successfully for thousands of years by Taoists trained through direct personal transmission from teacher to student. Readers should not undertake these practices without receiving personal transmission and training from a certified instructor of the Universal Healing Tao, since certain of these practices, if done improperly, may cause injury or result in health problems. This book is intended as a supplement to individual training in the Universal Healing Tao and as a reference guide for these practices. Anyone who undertakes these practices based on this book alone does so entirely at his or her own risk.

The meditations, practices, and techniques described herein are not intended to be used as an alternative or substitute for professional medical treatment and care. If any readers are suffering from an illness based on physical, mental, or emotional disorders, an appropriate professional health care practitioner or therapist should be consulted. Such problems should be addressed before you start Universal Healing Tao training.

The Universal Healing Tao staff and instructors are not responsible for the consequences of any practice or misuse of the information contained in this book. If the reader undertakes any exercise without strictly following the instructions, notes, and warnings, the responsibility lies solely with the reader.

This book does not attempt to give any medical diagnosis, treatment, prescription, or remedial recommendation in relation to any human disease, ailment, or physical condition whatsoever.

1

Addiction and Recovery from a Taoist Perspective

Imagine that this happens to you: You come home accompanied by a friend. You are surprised that some of your family members and other friends are already there waiting for you. One of them asks you to sit down with them in the circle they have made. Each of them takes a turn reading something they wrote. You are instructed that you are not allowed to respond until all of them have read what they have written. Each of their prepared statements expresses care and concern about your behavior. They are suggesting that you have an addiction. A lot of tears are shed, and the emotion in the room is thick.

This feels like an ambush and a betrayal to you. *How could they do this?* you ask yourself. You're thinking, *They're judging me and attacking me. This is unfair. I can stop whenever I want. I just like doing it. It's not a problem. I have great willpower. I can control myself. I can do whatever I want, it's my life. I know lots of people who do it more than me. They just don't understand . . .* They seem dead serious, though, threatening to stop helping you or even associating with you if you don't stop. How do you respond? What's the best way to handle this?

If you get mad or defensive, then you may lose them. *Maybe it's better to just play along*, you think.

ADDICTION DEFINED

What is addiction, anyway? It can be considered from different perspectives. The 12-Step community views it from a disease perspective. Gabor Maté, physician and addiction expert, has raised awareness of the value of viewing addiction as a trauma response. Psychologist Bruce Alexander has described addiction as the result of a chronic lack of connection in life. In his book *The Biology of Belief*, cell biologist and best-selling author Bruce Lipton describes how beliefs can be passed down through the generations, hence it seems possible that some of the beliefs that make people more vulnerable to trying or relying on addictive activities or substances could be the result of a predisposition that stems from the beliefs of previous generations. Other experts focus on the obsessive and compulsive aspects of addiction, while still others emphasize that addiction operates like a chronic condition such as diabetes or high blood pressure.

In our first book on addiction, *EMDR and the Universal Healing Tao: An Energy Approach to Overcoming Emotional Trauma*, Master Chia and Doug Hilton suggest that it is useful to view addiction as a response to adopting an overly yang lifestyle, which emphasizes and values extreme and aggressive tendencies, without enough of a yin approach to life to balance it out with gentleness, compassion, and letting go of what is not within our control. Examples of yang tendencies might be moving too quickly, relentlessly driving toward a desired goal without much consideration given to the process that it might take to reach it, and expending energy to reach the goal without taking adequate time to rest. Without referring to it in terms of yang or yin, the 12-Step community has long recognized that tendency and the need for a lifestyle change. They often use the term "Easy Does It" in their meetings. This is an important direction not just for people who have addictions; it also points to the change that is possible and indeed needed at the level of family, culture, and society if we wish to address the subtle and unconscious motivations behind addictive behavior. Effective prevention strategies need to address this, and not just give out information about the dangers of addiction.

In that first book we used Taoist concepts to point out the paradoxical nature of change and how adopting an overly yang lifestyle can lead to problems that lead to addictions. Being successful in life is often associated with ideas like being a go-getter, someone who "takes the bull by the horns" and "makes things happen." Putting effort into life is necessary to get results, of course, but too much aggression can lead to frustration and resentment—disturbed emotional states that are some of the building blocks for what can lead a person to turn to an addictive substance or activity in order to cope. In that book we suggested that the survival mechanisms that allow us to deny overwhelming circumstances so we can cope, forget our pain, and simply adapt may also be the mechanisms that can lead to addictive behavior. Addiction seems to exploit these human tendencies, leading us to gravitate to something unhealthy without realizing it.

As Gabor Maté and others have pointed out, trauma and the pileup of many unresolved feelings can also, consciously or unconsciously, push a person to find a powerful way to medicate those feelings. Being active in an addiction means that the normal way of processing emotions is not being allowed to function, so experiences that you would normally process and let go of become more difficult to resolve. As a result, the stuffed emotions pile up. And as more and more emotions get repressed, the need to self-medicate grows.

When people have experiences that shake their faith in themselves or whatever belief systems they have adopted, they become more vulnerable to addiction. If a sense of inner peace is not cultivated, then it will be only a matter of time before the person starts searching for substitutes for that peace.

Examining addiction from an energetic perspective, it becomes clear that the undigested emotions resulting from an addictive lifestyle will, like a clogged carburetor, block the energy flow in the channels and create an urgent need for the person to find something that can relieve them from their pain, even if only temporarily. The internal weight of those clogged emotions and the energy it takes to numb those painful emotions as much as possible drains a lot of energy. Addictive substances and activities may provide temporary relief, but they eventually plug up the internal channels even more, with toxic consequences as a result. If the internal processing system remains blocked for a long time and the "solutions" to address it are primarily addictive ones, new patterns that connect the problem feelings to addictive solutions become more solid over time. Since we are built to survive and to be internally consistent, eventually the internal core programming becomes permanently changed to accept the addictive solutions as necessary and required for proper functioning. Addiction prevention and recovery, from a Taoist perspective, involves keeping the energy channels open and clear or reopening and clearing them out again if there is a need to do so, so that the person can feel like they have space to deal with their life circumstances without having to resort to drastic measures to cope along the way.

THE CONSEQUENCES OF ADDICTION

The effects of addiction are many and varied. The virtues, or higher qualities, of the vital yin organs (the heart, the spleen, the lungs, the kidneys, the sexual organs, and the liver), which store physical, emotional, mental, and spiritual energy, become obscured by the buildup of toxicity. This translates into the addict looking and becoming older than their relative age would indicate, as their responses to life situations become more reactive and negative. As the energy channels that are connected to those yin organs become increasingly blocked over time with an overload of toxic energy, the result is chronic physical pain and a lack of well-being on all levels. The body's systems cry out for relief from the physical and emotional pain and demand that the substances or activities to which the person is addicted be provided. As a result, despite knowing better, people end up going back to their addictions in an attempt to give themselves relief from their symptoms.

When someone is actively engaged in feeding their addiction, they are not thinking as clearly and rationally as they would under normal circumstances. Their higher cognitive functions in the cerebral cortex are essentially hijacked and taken for a joyride. Addictions are progressive. They get worse the more the person feeds them, and it becomes harder and harder to stop. The yin organs then produce a variety of negative emotional states that lead to a personality of addiction that is named "Slick" in 12-Step meetings. This refers to the predictable combination of undesirable tendencies in addicts such as lying, manipulating, self-centeredness, and being impatient and demanding.*

Which approach to treating addiction is the correct one? All of them are correct to a certain extent, and none of them completely capture the mysterious nature of the problem enough to completely cure it. They all have value in terms of guiding treatment, and there are a few things they all agree on. They all recognize that addiction is not a problem of losers or a weak character. It is also generally accepted that addiction is not something that a person wants. All approaches agree that there is no way to know if someone will cross the line into addiction. It is also universally accepted that recovery from addiction is difficult and complicated. Consistent with Taoism, the focus of this book is not to attempt to draw lines of distinction to include some approaches and definitions and exclude others. The purpose is to instead take what

*Our book *EMDR and the Universal Healing Tao* offers a more detailed description of how depression, anxiety, and trauma tend to be linked to addiction, and how addictions develop.

is valuable from each perspective, blend it with the right ingredients from ancient knowledge, and integrate the different approaches so that an effective treatment can be created. It is difficult to imagine how a treatment approach of any kind could teach people how to embrace the reality of their lives and create positive outcomes if the approach is somehow based in judgment or an attitude of superiority.

HOW DO YOU KNOW IF YOU HAVE AN ADDICTION?

Defining addiction in terms of what you have been using, how much you use it, or how frequently you use it usually leads to debate. There is no magic number that defines a problem. It is usually more helpful and accurate to focus on the consequences and whether or not you have changed your lifestyle and created habits to accommodate the addictive substance or behavior. Be honest with yourself and answer these questions:

- Do the addictive thing(s) you use lead to or contribute to consequences that you don't want, like a hangover, arguments with loved ones, physical accidents, ignoring responsibilities, or debt?
- Do you continue to do something that is potentially addictive despite the consequences? Put your pride aside and answer this question. If you are not dependent on that thing, why are you so determined to hold onto it?
- Think about this one: When you were a kid thinking about your future, is this what you hoped it would be? Is this the ideal that you have been hoping to reach?
- How much time in your day do you spend planning around that addictive thing? How much time do you spend actually doing it or using it? Would you think it was okay if someone else was doing what you're doing?

TYPES OF ALCOHOLISM

Addiction to alcohol can be tricky to define. There is more than one type of addiction to alcohol. There are three types, in fact. One type is the one that most people picture when the word *alcoholic* is mentioned. They think of someone who is drunk pretty much every day and is obviously inebriated. That type of alcoholic cannot function well enough to stay on top of her or his daily responsibilities. The image of someone lying in a gutter on the street, wearing dirty clothes, in need of a shower, and clutching a paper bag with bottle concealed in it comes to mind. Another, less-known type is what is referred to as a *binge alcoholic*. This person may not drink often, but when he or she does drink it is almost always to excess, whether that was the intention of the person at the outset or not. This type is trickier to accept as an addiction because the person is able to abstain for extended periods of time. Again, it is the consequences, the lack of control, and the compulsion to continue despite those consequences that defines it as a problem. The third type—also difficult to reconcile as a problem—is called *maintenance alcoholism*. This describes a pattern in which the person drinks regularly, often daily, but does not usually appear drunk. People who have this type of alcoholism are called functional alcoholics. This person can still manage their daily responsibilities, but the problem is that the person needs those few drinks, and the long-term effects of regular drinking can be as severe as the other types.

CODEPENDENCY

Addiction does not just affect the person who is afflicted. It also affects the people closest to them as well. People who are in regular contact with someone who is in active addiction tend to develop predictable patterns of responding to them that soon become predictable patterns of responding to life in general. The two most common patterns are trying to control that which is out of their control, and the tendency to worry. It is natural for people to develop those tendencies under the circumstances—someone they love is clearly in danger and they cannot make them realize that. In a sense, the loved ones develop addictive behavior just like the afflicted person, but their focus is on the person and her or his condition rather than on an addictive substance or activity. The term that is commonly attached to this type of pattern is *codependency*.

Codependency refers to the tendency for a person to do things for another person that they could or should do for themselves and to focus more on the needs of others than on their own needs. These tendencies can remain long after the person who has the addiction has stopped. The triggers for people who have an addiction are the people, places, things, and situations that remind them of their addiction; the triggers for people who struggle with codependency are the people who have addictions themselves and anything or anyone who reminds them of their addicted loved one.

There can be a lot of conflict between the person in recovery and their loved ones because of the codependency issue. The person with an addiction wants and needs freedom to work through their recovery. Their friends or family worry that they might relapse, so they try to control their behavior so they themselves can stop worrying. The person in recovery resents being controlled like this, and their defensiveness and resentment only serve to confirm the worries of their family and friends. Power struggles can develop, and conflict can easily escalate to the point where marriages, family connections, and friendships can be destroyed by such struggles.

The practices in this book can benefit anyone no matter which side of the fence you're on. If you have a codependency pattern, the more you practice, the better you will become at meeting your own needs without having to control other people and situations around you. It is more productive and effective to work on oneself than to try to change the mind and behavior of someone we love. Then happiness does not depend on what they do or do not do. The ideal situation is when everyone who is directly or indirectly affected by an addiction uses the practices in this book regularly.

THE TAOIST APPROACH

Taoism is an ancient spiritual philosophy that examines the natural laws of life and how to live in harmony with nature. Taoism does not require people to change or accept new truths about the existence of God or particular gods, about what happens after we die, and what we should or should not do while we are alive. Taoism only comments on the dynamics of nature and how we can move in harmony with those dynamics if we so choose. As a result, people who do not embrace a particular religious faith as well as those who do can both enjoy learning about Taoism without having to sacrifice their spiritual beliefs or nonbeliefs.

Taoism provides an energetic framework that teaches people how to flow with life. The Universal Healing Tao system in particular offers practical applications of ancient Taoist concepts. The practices in this book were highly guarded secrets for millennia before Master Chia started to share them with the world. This book provides step-by-step instructions from different Chi Kung practices in the Universal Healing Tao system as well as clear explanations as to how the practices relate to addiction recovery. Read this book to learn how to open the energy channels in your body and mind, circulate that energy, and thereby clean, balance, and strengthen your energy without any artificial aids. Learn how to use your mind and body together to direct your future toward health and happiness.

Before we go into the Taoist practices highlighted in this book, it's important to understand two foundational terms from this approach:

- **Chi** is the bioelectromagnetic energy in our bodies as well as the electromagnetic energy found all around us. It is known by other names, such as *prana*, *mana*, *ki*, *qi*, *elixir*, and *ether*. In our bodies it's what gives us life. All healing traditions agree that we have it within us.
- **Chi Kung** essentially translates as "energy work." It refers to the practice of deliberately mastering the mind, body, and breath to harness the power of our chi and to use it to increase our health and happiness. Some people define Chi Kung as "mastering the breath." Chi Kung includes practices that are done seated, standing, lying down, and moving. Chi Kung can also be used for healing others, both with touch and without touch. Chi Kung uses the mind, movement, colors, and sounds to access the proper energy frequencies for our well-being. It can also involve directing the mind to access specific energies from certain directions, forces, and elements.

The aim of Chi Kung is to increase the general sense of well-being of a person so that he or she can then address all of their problems more effectively. The belief is that the body and mind can heal themselves if there is enough healing energy circulating freely through the person. It teaches people how to make themselves healthy by learning how to move chi through all of the meridians (energy channels) in the body, through practices that are done while seated, standing, moving, and lying down. The tools that are taught are called "practices" because that is what is required to make them work—practice! The instructors do not claim to be the source of the healing that is provided; they simply teach people *how* to create health. Energy work is enjoyable. It can be fun. It seems logical that participants will be more likely to continue to use what they have learned in their treatment experience for an addiction if they enjoy what they are doing. Taoist practices do not require great flexibility, strength, or coordination, nor do they require expensive clothing or equipment. The only requirements are that the person wears comfortable clothing and has a small, open space in which to practice.

Keep in mind that one of the goals of recovery from the Taoist perspective is to create a personalized and flexible routine of healthy activities that is short, simple, and portable, but comprehensive enough to keep you on track. The benefit of having a regular routine is that if you practice it faithfully, then eventually it becomes somewhat automatic, to the point where it feels like something is missing if you do not do it. The idea is that if it eventually becomes as automatic as brushing your teeth, then you might do it even when your mind is a bit foggy about why it is so important to do it. We all go up and down in our motivation and it is difficult to maintain a routine forever. If you want proof of that, just go to your local gym right after New Year's Eve. It will be packed. Three or four weeks later it is not nearly so packed. We are built to forget pain. That is one of our survival mechanisms. Therefore it's easy to get complacent and start thinking, *Oh, I don't feel like it today. Missing one day won't be such a big deal. I'm better now. I don't need to be so careful. I was probably just going through a rough patch before.* Denial comes in like clouds in the sky. Pick the practices that you enjoy the most or need the most and make a routine for yourself. Change it if you need to, but do not stop practicing.

Many people who have successfully stopped using their addictive substances or activities will start to have the desire to help others do the same. This is natural and a good thing. Many addiction counselors have ended up in their field after first stopping their own addictions. The twelfth step in the 12-Step program is about helping others as a part of the recovery process. Having personal experience with addiction and recovery can help you understand how difficult the process can be. People who are struggling in their recovery can feel comforted by hearing that you have "been there and done that."

However, there are some important concepts to keep in mind as you proceed on your journey of helping others with their addictions. To start with, helping people can be far more complicated than it seems at first. Although there are common themes in addiction and recovery, everyone has a unique personality and a unique story. We are affected by each person differently as well. As a result, personal experience with the process does not necessarily mean that your own experience will be sufficient to guide you in helping someone else. Another important idea to remember is to make sure that you create as much space inside yourself as possible before trying to be there for someone else. If you have an addiction of your own, even if you have chalked up years of recovery, getting too drained or overloaded by the challenges that someone else has might trigger you to go back to your addiction. Training in the Universal Healing Tao system can help you to be as prepared and safe on your path of helping others as possible.

As well, keep in mind that it is very useful to have personally experienced the effects of the practices that you are going to introduce to someone else. It is also important to remember that helping others is a process that needs to be approached at the right time and in the right way. Otherwise it is possible to end up using the idea of helping others as another quick fix that you are using to replace the addiction that you are trying to manage in yourself. If you are going to be an effective coach, sponsor, or counselor, you need to be able to put your personal needs aside and focus on helping the people that you are trying to serve.

Lastly, people who receive help from someone can usually tell if the person is not sincere or is not wholeheartedly involved in the process of helping. Maintaining your own routine of Universal Healing Tao practices can help you to reach out to others in a sincere and heartfelt manner.

2

What Is Recovery?

Recovery is a term that is commonly used to describe what people are supposed to aim for and achieve when they deal with their addictions. What does it mean, though? Many people in early recovery assume that it means to just stop using what feeds their addiction. Later on in recovery they usually learn that recovery requires changing one's habits and lifestyle and creating healthier habits and a better balance in one's life. Upon further contemplation, these notions bring up a host of other questions:

- What is included in a balanced lifestyle?
- How do I know how much of a particular balance is the right amount for me?
- Who gets to set the standards for my lifestyle? My family? Society?
- How much is healthy enough or balanced enough?
- Is recovery just about getting my old life back that I had before I developed an addiction?
- Do I have to figure out some root problem that caused my addiction and learn how to manage it?
- What do things like self-esteem, happiness, and religion or spirituality have to do with recovery?

The truth is that there is no consensus regarding the answers to these questions. Different programs and practitioners will offer varying opinions and guidance. People who have addictions often have a history of broken trust, and so they have difficulty trusting even in the best of times. They can often sense that what they are being offered in treatment settings is not the only truth that they could consider. That makes it difficult for them to embrace what they are being offered. Some of them attend multiple treatment programs before they are able to stabilize their recovery. If the guidance they receive in each setting is different, it can become very difficult to know what is best and to commit to that approach with the kind of dedication that it takes to achieve long-term recovery. They can also have difficulty accepting the program that they are being offered if it does not meet the needs they know they must address. It is very difficult for a single program to meet *all* of the needs of participants. Therefore, most programs end up making decisions about what they can and cannot include in their program. For example, areas that are often left unaddressed in most treatment programs involve trauma, how to increase participants' connection to themselves and others, and self-regulation of one's emotional states.

Thankfully, people like Gabor Maté have highlighted the need to address trauma as an important factor in the successful treatment of addictions. It seems like this perspective is gaining traction in the treatment field. However, in order to more completely address trauma it's crucial that we look at our society and how it creates trauma. Modern society focuses too much on the accumulation of wealth and things and not enough on how to feel at peace without them or on how to make sure that we do not use up too much energy in the pursuit of those things. If a person goes for professional help to stop engaging in an addiction but returns after treatment to a lifestyle based on "more is better" or "whoever dies with the most toys wins," then they are bound to experience frustration and resentment when life makes it difficult to get what they want. And this can be the trigger that takes the person right back into their addiction.

To give addiction recovery its proper and deserved position in society it might be important to first recognize how a broken society promotes addiction. Governments have relied on revenue from cigarettes, alcohol, and gambling for many decades. The medical system is overwhelmed and overwhelming, and relies heavily on medicating symptoms with pharmaceutical drugs. Never-ending wars continue, and weapons have become more lethal. Natural disasters are happening more frequently and are getting worse, and the subject of weather manipulation has entered the mainstream conversation. The financial situation of many ordinary people is precarious, with many not having any money set aside for emergencies. The media focuses on the most dire news to amp up fear, anger, and a sense of helplessness. It's no wonder that so many people find themselves self-medicating.

The accumulation of all of these stresses of modern life can have the same triggering effect as a single overwhelming traumatic event. The emotional weight of these stresses accumulates like grains of sand in an hourglass until the whole way of operating is flipped upside down. Addiction treatment therefore needs to teach people how to handle the steady accumulation of negative emotions as they go through life, so they do not build up to the point where a person needs to medicate them.

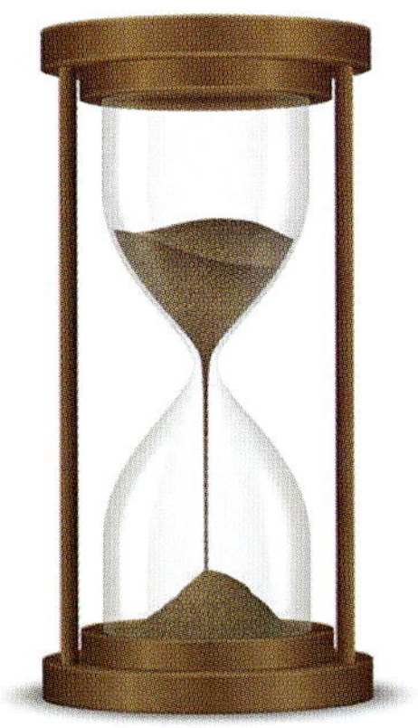

Fig. 2.1. Small events can lead to big problems.

It is important to realize that we do not have unlimited energy. When we use up too much of it we tend to panic and resort to extreme measures to regain it, similar to how people tend to panic if they suddenly realize that their car is almost out of gas, so they rush to the nearest gas station to fill up. For people who have an addiction, that is a dangerous way to meet their needs. It creates a momentum that involves quick fixes, drama, and chaos. The more people approach life that way, the more likely it is they will eventually consider feeding their addiction as an easy way to deal with their next crisis. That is why recovery often involves cleaning up the messes that have been created while the person was in active addiction.

There are many surprises and complications that occur in the process of recovery, so it's no wonder people trying to address their addictions are often overwhelmed. Treatment programs frequently leave out or underrepresent treatment of trauma because of the amount of time it would take to provide proper support and the uncertainty around which kinds of trauma treatment will work best for clients. Those providers who specialize in self-regulation training, which involves control of one's thoughts, emotions, and behaviors, often do not have much specific training in addiction treatment, and though many treatment

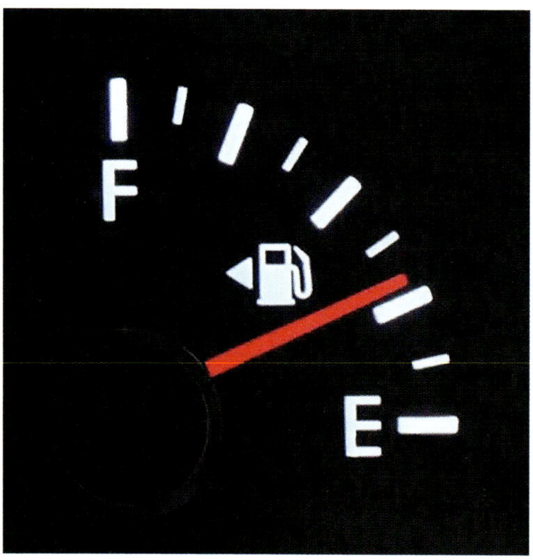

Fig. 2.2. Emptying more than filling leads to panic and quick fixes.

programs do offer a component that touches on self-control, it usually falls short of what's needed. A comprehensive addiction treatment program thus needs to teach people how to build, monitor, and protect their energy and to regulate their emotions so they are not so easily overwhelmed by life events.

How a person feels about their life, their purpose, and their community is an important determinant in creating a life that is more fulfilling and worthwhile than when that person was in active addiction. Like anyone else would be, but often to a greater degree among addicts, those who seek treatment are not comfortable being told what to believe about their life and their place in it. This makes addressing those issues challenging in treatment. Effective and thorough treatment of addiction requires finding ways to talk about spirituality without forcing a particular belief system on clients.

TREATMENT OPTIONS

What happens when a person agrees to go for treatment? When most people think about addiction treatment, they think "rehab". People who have never been inside a rehab facility often do not have much information about what might happen there. To most people, rehab is some kind of big black box in which people go in and come out weeks or months later seemingly dramatically changed, like they went through some kind of washing machine for people with addictions. Although rehab is definitely one of the types of environments that is offered, it is not the only one.

Rehab refers to what is also called intensive residential treatment. This type of treatment option requires participants to live on the premises with a number of other people with addictions for at least twenty-eight days. There is frequent interaction with counselors every day, mostly in group formats. Some programs are only for one sex, some are based on the 12-Step program, while others are not. By living on-site,

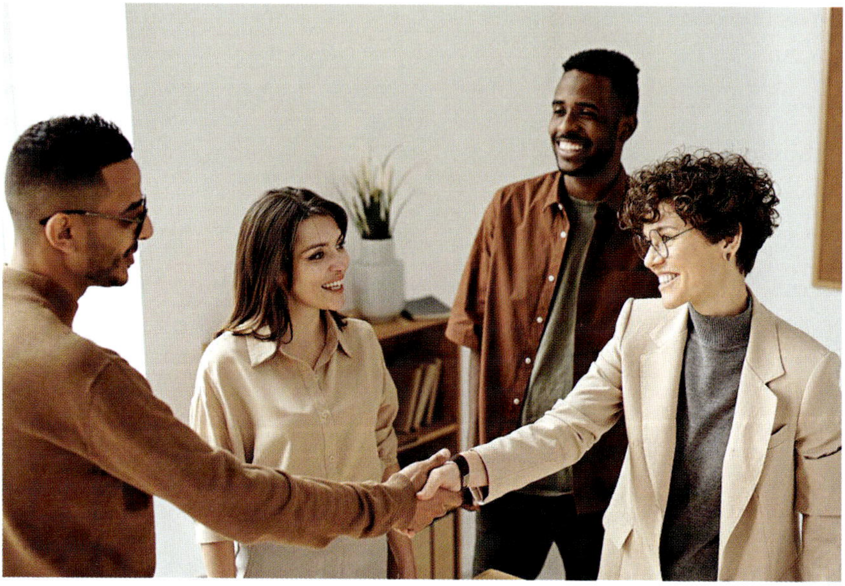

Fig. 2.3. Walking into a building and being greeted by a friendly face.

those in rehab are able to stay away from many of their triggering people, places, and situations for a specific period of time. Day treatment is a similar model except that participants do not live on-site. Supportive recovery or recovery houses do require participants to live on-site, but the treatment interaction with counselors is not usually as frequent or as extensive as it is in residential or day treatment programs.

Outpatient treatment involves attending counseling sessions, individual as well as group sessions in some places, on a periodic basis. Clients might attend sessions at an outpatient treatment facility a few times a week at most. Detox, or "withdrawal management" as it is known, is primarily focused on helping people who have addictions to alcohol or drugs to safely get those chemicals out of their systems. Participants stay on-site and are monitored by medical professionals until they have completed the detox process and are healthy enough to leave.

Each type of program has a mandate, often accompanied by guidelines or limits for how long a person can continue to receive treatment there. They also usually have particular aspects of treatment that they focus on. For example, simply due to the fact that residential treatment programs have a standard format and a standard duration, they often are not able to completely treat underlying trauma issues. Many outpatient clinics have the same kinds of constraints as well. As a result, people are often referred between many services because none of them are fully equipped or even allowed to address all of the issues involved. Due to the narrow view of some aspects of the recovery model, addiction is not addressed fully even if the person is willing to jump through all of the hoops to access the various services. Detoxification is an example. In most programs, detoxing refers to the process of drying out so that the substances that the person has been using are not noticeably still in their system. That's a good idea. It helps the person readjust to how it feels to be clean and sober. However, detoxifying is something that we all do on a regular basis. We all collect toxins from various sources—the air we breathe, the food we eat, and the emotions we experience. Teaching people how to do energetic exercises that help them consciously clean their systems out allows them to reduce their level of toxicity on a regular basis. Detoxification, like recovery, is a process, not a single event.

12-Step programs like Alcoholics Anonymous (AA) and Narcotics Anonymous have been around for almost a century. They are run by volunteers and are found all over the world. AA is abstinence-based, meaning that the goal of attending the meetings is to stop using an addictive substance and stay away from it. Like anything else, these programs have mixed reviews. Some people love the meetings and view them as key to their recovery. Some people view AA as a cult because participants repeat certain phrases as a group and because the terms *God* and *Higher Power* are used in the meetings. Those terms are meant to refer to whatever each participant believes in, though. That is the only part of the written twelve steps that is written in bold. If people are going to try 12-Step meetings, it's usually a good idea to try to experience a few different meetings and reserve any judgments based on initial impressions.

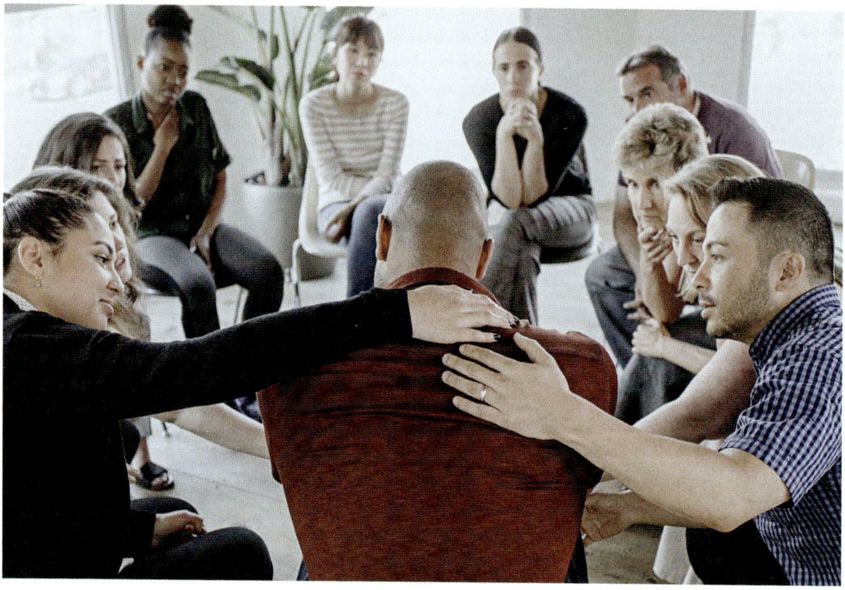

Fig. 2.4. You cannot do it alone.

A SYSTEM IN NEED OF REBALANCING

Addiction recovery is hard to maintain. There are hundreds of dedicated professionals in the addiction recovery field who work hard to help. Many clients will testify that the treatment and support they received from the various components of addiction treatment saved their lives. However, many clients still relapse within a week after completing a treatment program. It is the responsibility of the field of addictions treatment to continue striving to improve. Addictions treatment programs have developed, expanded, and evolved to the point where some of the limitations to the directions in which they seem to be headed have become clear.

Most addiction treatment programs lean heavily on information about how the person can use their mind to stay clearheaded about the reality of their addictive problem. This means they must focus on strategies to stay away from the ideas, situations, people, and behaviors that will eventually lead them back to their addictive substance or behavior.

Symptoms are assessed, and then specific concepts, information, and strategies are offered to address them. This is a necessary and important part of addiction treatment and recovery.

Again, the purpose of this book is not to criticize other approaches that have helped people. The intent, instead, is to highlight the need for energetic approaches to supplement existing treatment approaches for greater benefit and lasting results. Without an energetic approach to treatment, people may end up playing whack-a-mole with their symptoms, using sheer willpower to try to stay a step ahead of their addictive thoughts or urges. The treatment ends up being symptom management through thinking as a substitute for using. This approach can be exhausting and frustrating. Addiction affects the automatic aspect of the nervous system. It can affect a person despite her or his best intentions, and it is not ruled by willpower. Blinking, an activity that is managed by the automatic part of the nervous system, illustrates why this is so. Imagine that you decided to use your willpower and self-awareness to stop blinking or to blink less often. Realistically, how long could you

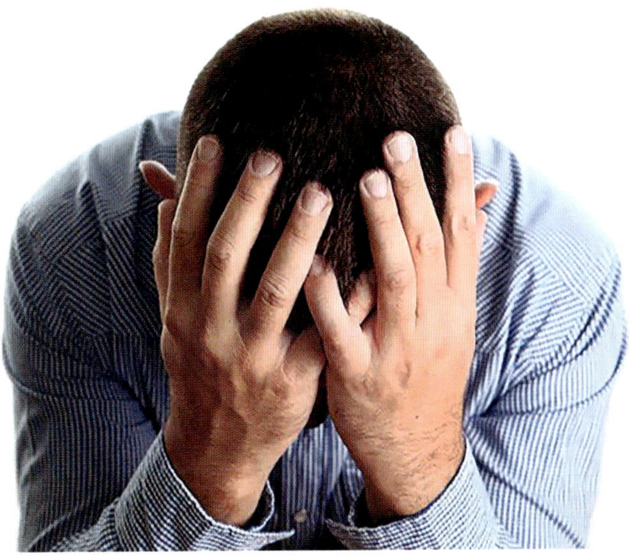

Fig. 2.5. Try not to overthink it.

manage that? Not long. It's not because of your lack of intelligence, willpower, or moral fiber.

Another consequence of addressing addiction using strategies that mostly involve thinking is that this can result in the seemingly endless task of identifying innumerable subcategories of problems to be addressed, such as behavioral issues, neurodivergent categories, learning disabilities, personality disorders, and psychiatric conditions. If you put the power to recover in the hands of the so-called professionals, then you need paperwork and policies to police their conduct to make sure they are treating people the best way possible. The more we learn about all the historical, emotional, and cognitive aspects behind each person's addiction, the more problems we seem to need to address. In this model, each and every one of the endless number of triggering people, places, and things that could cause a person to return to an addiction needs to be addressed so that the person can stay on track. Cognitive approaches like this operate using analysis, often breaking the problem down with deductive reasoning. This basically mental approach tends to ask, "What is the problem?" followed by "Why has this happened?" then "What are the obstacles to solving the problem?" and finally "What are the options for addressing the problem?" Energetic approaches as found in Taoism, in contrast, simply teach people how to make themselves feel better, regardless of whichever treatment model they follow.

From an administrative standpoint, cognitive treatment approaches that emphasize managing symptoms involve a long list of policies and procedures to make sure that clients stay protected from harm and that the treatment facility is legally protected from liability. In all career fields there are people who have good intentions and those who do not. An unfortunate reality that is frequently a byproduct of treatment centers that emphasize a specific model of thinking strategies is that such facilities tend to attract employees who want to take credit for the power of their approach and so they may try to control others to protect their viewpoint. Systems with lots of bureaucracy (government-funded ser-

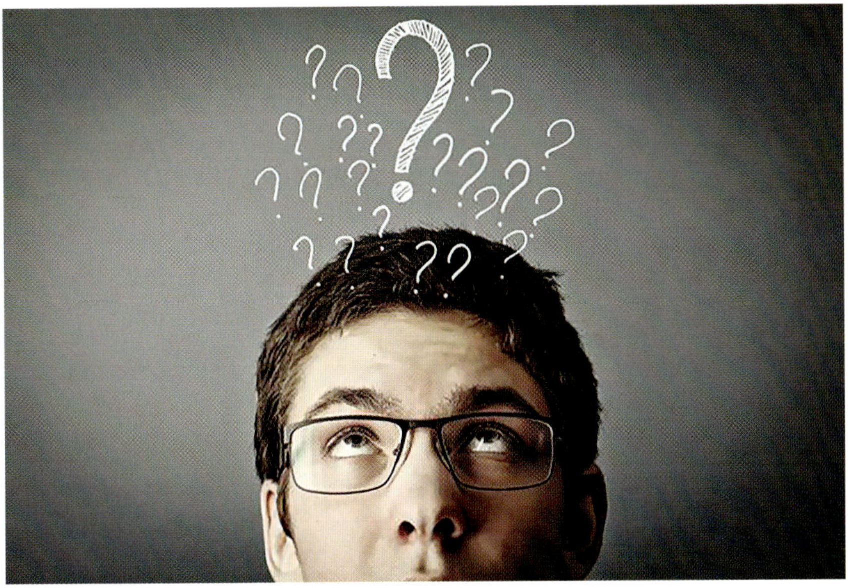

Fig. 2.6. Why? How? When? Where? What now?

vices are a good example) can attract administrators who seek power, as well as impostors, incompetents, and even sociopaths and psychopaths. They can hide and flourish in these kinds of settings through double-talk, bullying, and harassment. They create empires to rule in which they vilify their staff and create ever-increasing levels of administration to maintain control. This results in a system that reinforces itself. The emphasis is on finding noncompliance with the new rules while creating more and more rules. The result is a program that is supposed to be teaching clients how to focus on the recovery process but instead is focused on results at the administrative level. Such a system needs to keep identifying new battles to fight in order to justify its existence. To identify new battles to fight, these systems need to keep analyzing and dissecting the "helping" process to identify what needs to be micromanaged next. Imagine how much money it takes to pay for all of that.

There is money, status, and power attached to creating or aligning with a model of treatment or of outcome monitoring. Models of service delivery are popping up in the counseling field that are being forced on counselors through policies and procedures in a similar manner to how cults have forced their followers to adhere to a particular way of living. Punitive consequences follow if a counselor questions the creators of the models or the model itself. If you want a clue as to whether or not a cult mentality is connected to your treatment program, check to see if negative feedback exists for it on the internet. If there is none, it is probably because someone is making sure of that. All models receive criticism at some point. Another clue is if there are no formal ways for recourse if the model is used as a weapon by management in a service to harass or bully staff or contractors.

Evidence-based is the current buzz term that is often used to justify taking particular approaches to addictions treatment. It usually refers to using quantitative research results to decide what does and does not work. It assumes that research results from controlled circumstances are more accurate than observation in natural environments, that statistical results (especially ones that are found more than once) are indisputable truth, and that they are more objective than the opinions or observations of counselors. It is important to remember that research can be manipulated, too, and that it is affected by the biases of the researchers. It is also true that, with the amount of research data that has been compiled to date, a person can find research results to back up almost any opinion about what treatments work best. The treatment and outcome measurement cults seem to rely heavily on that fact. They gather research results that fit their ideology, or results that they can interpret in a way that fits it, and then offer them as proof that their approach is the truth or the best.

Evidence that a treatment program is being administered by people who are too unhealthy or unethical can be found in actions like making vague threats toward the staff ("I'm going to be cutting your pay. I'll let you know how much later"); referring to staff like they are just numbers to be added or deleted as needed ("I got a new assistant. We moved some money around"); making unilateral decisions but then blaming the staff if they get caught doing the same; creating more and more policies and procedures until even the most well-meaning staff cannot keep up with them, and then labeling their inability to keep up as "rebellious"; making verbal promises and then refusing to honor them; "benching" staff by refusing any requests they make to offer a new contribution to the service; and having people sign nondisclosure agreements to keep their positions so they cannot voice their concerns in public.

The counselors in these kinds of systems are not usually entirely innocent in these dynamics, either. They are often people who have addiction histories themselves, and so they usually have their own past issues with authority and do not like being told what to do. In addition, there are hundreds of recognized approaches to therapy, and counselors often devote a lot of time and effort to getting trained to determine which approaches suit them best. After all of that time and effort, they are usually not very open to having their boss tell them how to do their work. Such an approach to addictions treatment requires a lot of structure and compliance with that structure, so a fair amount of the treatment experience can be taken up with discussions about what to do about people who are not complying, since people with addictions often have historical issues with authority and struggle with a lack of self-discipline.

For all of these reasons, confidential evaluations need to be conducted regularly to prevent treatment programs from getting to these extremes. Checks and balances need to be a formal aspect of treatment programs so that ethical and fair practices can be restored if need be.

It would be unfair to suggest that all treatment programs only focus on information and strategies. There are many treatment services that teach their clients more than just how to think differently to manage their addictions. For example, many studies have shown

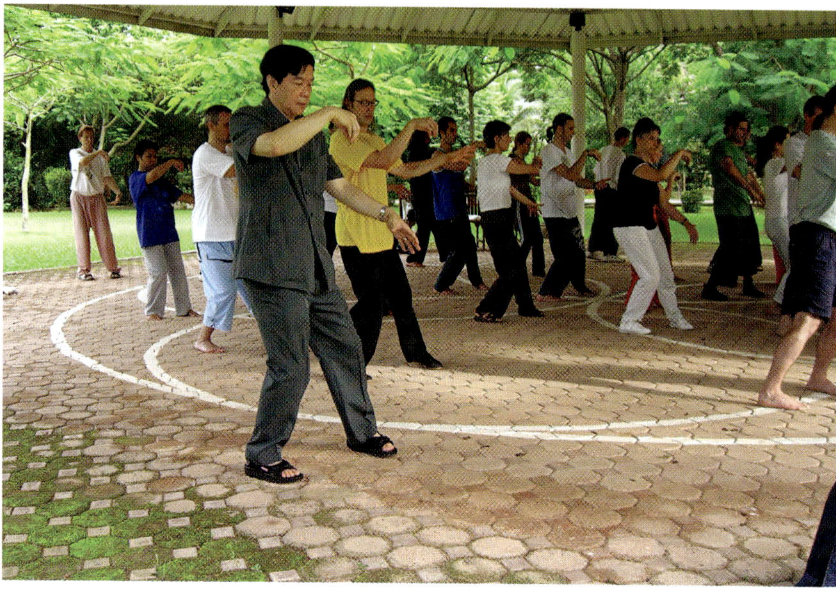

Fig. 2.7. Chi Kung is an energy-based practice, something missing in many treatment programs. Chi Kung in the Tai Chi Field at Tao Garden.

that the acupuncture protocol for treating addictive urges is effective, so it has been included in treatment services in both private and government-funded programs. Many residential programs include yoga and meditation. The 12-Step community has always recognized that their program works best when it is combined with prayer and meditation. However, the important piece that is missing, we feel, is the inclusion of energy-based practices to address the specific challenges in recovery that are not addressed in other ways.

THE WAY OF HARMONY AND BALANCE

At this point it is probably obvious that addiction treatment is more complicated than it seems on the surface. To find a system of treatment that does not claim to have answers about the ultimate truths in life and teaches people how to apply the generally accepted concepts in recovery

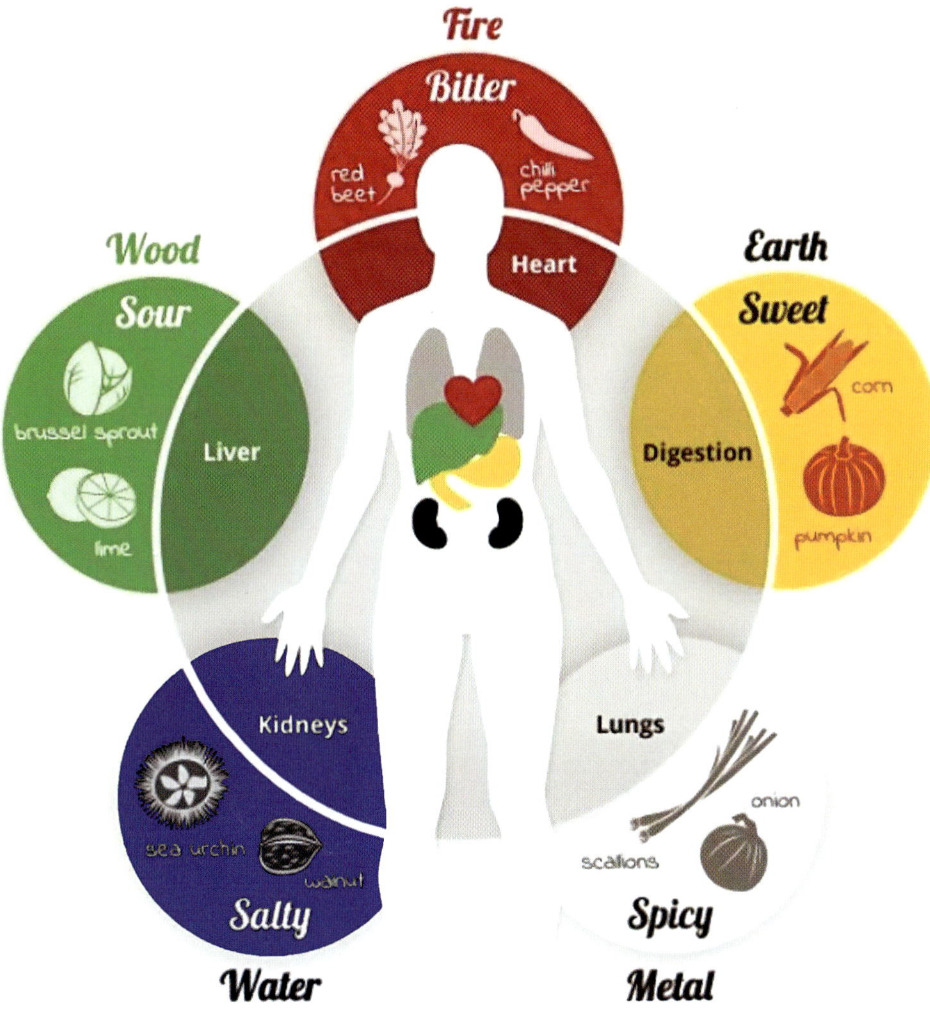

Fig. 2.8. The intrinsic connection between the elements, colors, sounds, and forces is a hallmark of Taoism.

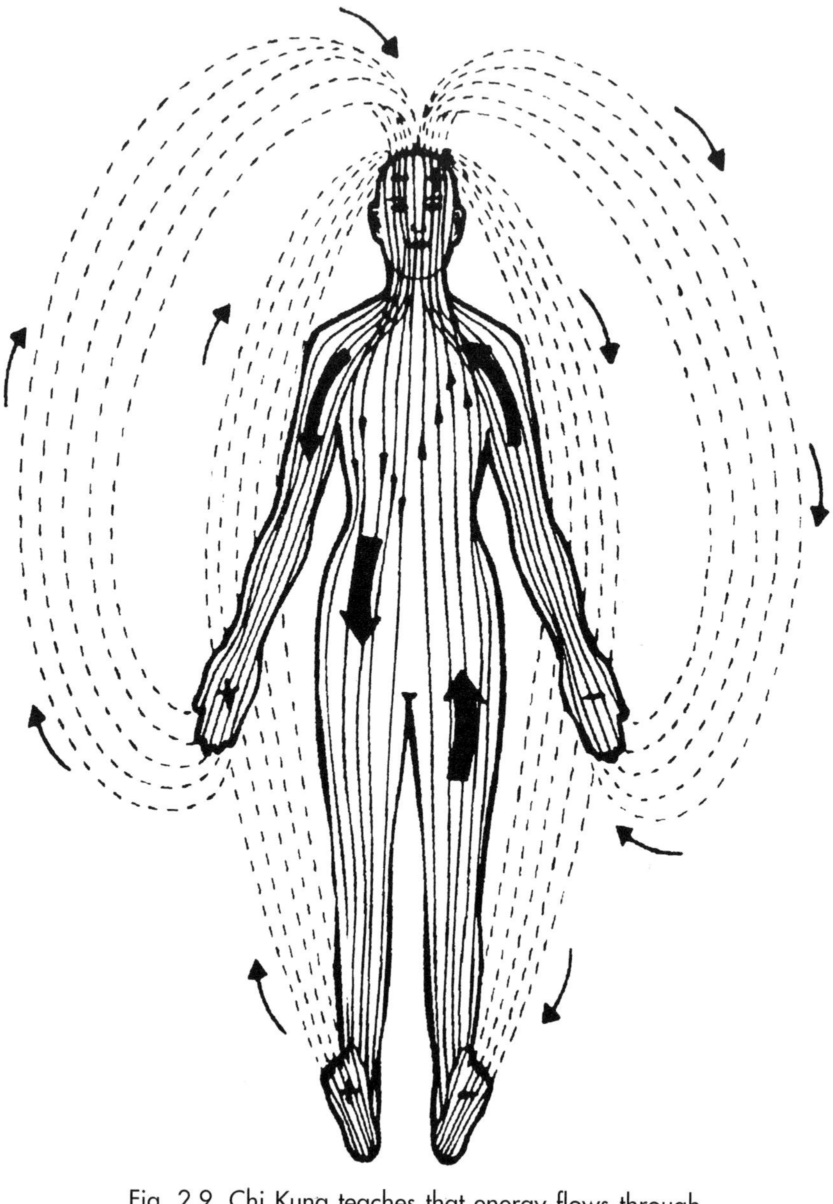

Fig. 2.9. Chi Kung teaches that energy flows through the body like rivers and streams.

in ways that they can enjoy according to their individual preferences seems like a tall order.

Taoism can fill that order. For some people, hearing the word *Taoism* might bring up preconceived ideas about an Asian religion that worships gods they have never heard of. Actually, Taoism focuses on how a balance in nature is achieved and maintained, and its practices bring the body, mind, and spirit in alignment with nature. There are no specific gods that need to be worshipped, no theories about the meaning of life or about what happens after we die. In fact, the only requirement is that we must practice.

Taoist concepts can be applied to food and home décor, as well as to physical, mental, emotional, and spiritual health. Chi Kung, meaning "energy work," one of the principal areas of the application of Taoism, offers methods for achieving internal balance in terms of colors, sounds, directions, elements, and types of forces. Chi Kung teaches us about the natural world within us and how to keep things flowing through all of the body's rivers and streams of energy. It emphasizes yin over yang (building and restoring energy over expending it), remaining humble, letting go of striving in order to feel peaceful, avoiding inviting jealousy and attack from others, and placing less emphasis on accumulating material things as a means to happiness.

The following excerpts are from Lao Tzu's Tao Te Ching as translated by Edward Brennan and Tao Huang, and published in *The Secret Teachings of the Tao Te Ching*.

Esteem is rooted in the humble.
The high is founded upon the low.
This is why the lords and rulers call themselves widows
and orphans without support.
Is this not the root of being humble?
Much praise amounts to no praise. (39: 4-6)

There are a lot of advantages to thinking about, talking about, and working on our energy. First of all, we're referring to an element of the human experience to which we can all relate, regardless of age, culture, or socioeconomic status. If someone says they feel "weighed down" by a problem in their life, for example, we all have some sense of what that means. When two people meet and feel romantically attracted to each other, we say there is a "spark" or "electricity" between them. When someone is tired and overwhelmed, we often use terms like *fried*, *frazzled*, or *burned out*. Why do we speak like this? Because these terms express how we *feel*. We know what our experience is. The language of energy bridges people from all walks of life. It also lifts the status of some cultures and cultural practices that were previously viewed as primitive to a level that is more on par with the rest of the world. Energy practices can be enjoyed by anyone. The experiences that people have when they perform the practices are unique and different for everyone. People whose personalities, preferences, and lifestyles cannot easily conform to an artificial system can have a place to fit, belong, and feel a connection. Ironically, most people who have addictions have an adverse reaction to the medications that are so often prescribed. And despite the impression you may have from watching 12-Step meetings acted out on television and in the movies, a lot of people with addiction issues may not like participating in group situations. Chi Kung is something that people can learn and practice on their own if they so choose.

Doing energy work does not have to mean rejecting mainstream society or its offerings. Ideally, people who practice Chi Kung live in the modern world but maintain their awareness of the energy world *at the same time*, so they can still function and benefit from the upsides of both. Learning how to master one's energy can be viewed as a potential new world of spirituality. By increasing their health and sense of well-being on all levels, people can be less reliant on government, spouses, family members, doctors, and other professionals to fix their problems for them. Then those people, institutions, and services become more of a bonus than a requirement. Hopefully one day our society will become more focused on rewarding people for learning how to heal and take better care of themselves. That will likely work better than punishing them for not doing those things.

Energy work has different guiding principles than those that underlie the Western medical system, which sees the body as consisting of discrete, unrelated material elements. Working with energy allows your muscles to soften as you focus on all aspects of your being—physical, mental, and emotional; you feel good without having to resort to extreme measures. Chi Kung practices help you soften and loosen your body and open the energy channels to circulate the life force. In Chi Kung we emulate the way water moves through a stream or the way a gentle breeze moves through the air. It's a lifestyle, not just an activity. The practices do not prescribe anything. They merely point the way back to our own individual balance. When we practice energy work, we feel peaceful inside and will likely feel less of a need to exploit opportunities to the detriment of others. When peace is created on the inside, there is less of a desire for people to engage in wars outside. This makes Taoism and its practices a great fit for people who are dealing with addictions.

3

The Chi Kung Approach

When it comes to addiction treatment there are notable differences between the Taoist approach and the typical Western approach. Both the Western and Chi Kung perspectives acknowledge that there is no consensus about what an addiction is, but the Chi Kung approach says that what is immaterial becomes material. In other words, the emotional and chemical changes in a person, whether naturally or artificially induced, will eventually become something denser and more solid, therefore more resistant to change.

The typical Western perspective on addiction is that people who have addictions suffer from some sort of defect of character as a result of bad habits that have been repeated too many times. Therefore, the person in treatment needs to keep track of those supposed defects and try to remove them by developing new habits or through appeals to a Higher Power. Chi Kung, on the other hand, operates from the belief that our internal organs can produce positive or negative emotions depending on what the person has experienced, what kinds of toxins they've been exposed to, and what their original constitution is from birth. The goal in Chi Kung is to learn how to transform the negative emotions into positive ones.

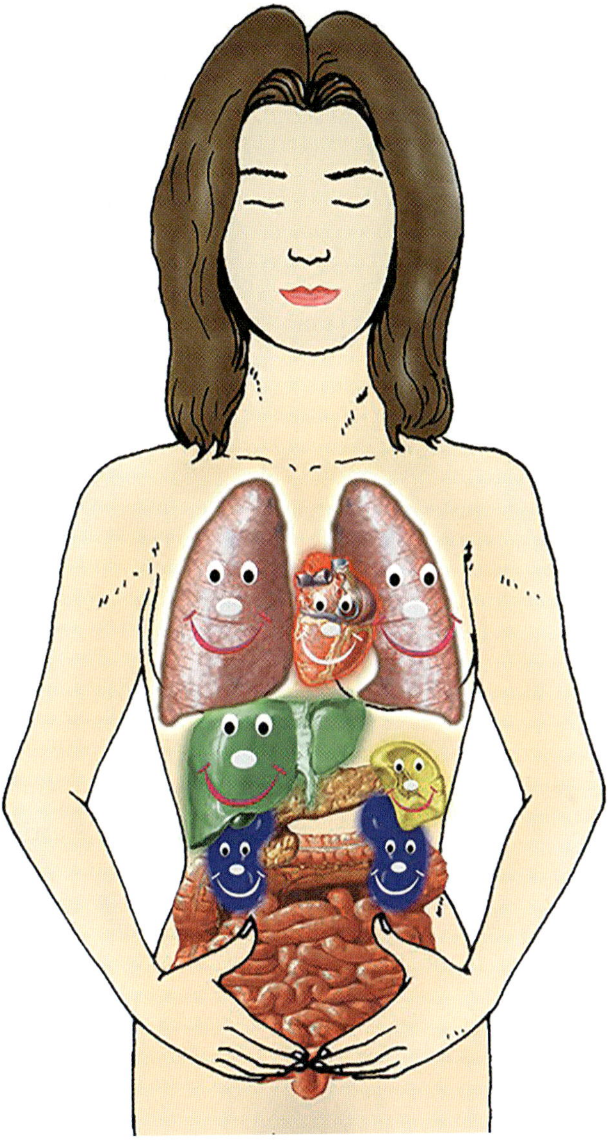

Fig. 3.1. Connections between elements of the body's organs.

The common Western perspective offered in addiction treatment is that people should try to solve their problems as best they can, but then they should "let go and let God." The concept of a Higher Power is not suggested in all treatment programs, but for the programs that do incorporate this concept it often becomes an intellectual stumbling block for many clients. It is not uncommon for people in treatment to envision that there is some old guy with a gray beard sitting on a throne in the sky, watching and judging. Of course, that is not the intention behind that suggestion, but it still poses a challenge for those who reject the concept of a patriarchal God. Optimism and faith, including faith in a Higher Power, are also difficult for them because they usually have seen life fall apart at various times in their past. The aim of Taoist Chi Kung practices is different—we say that people should learn to go with the flow of life as much as possible, to get out of their heads about what life is supposed to be like and realize that there is energy all around us and within us that can be used to help us feel better regardless of whether or not our problems can be solved.

Another difference: The Western approach prioritizes thinking strategies as the principal way to manage addictions, and prayer and meditation are added at some point later to help people regulate their emotions along the way. The thinking aspect of recovery is of course necessary, but it can be hard work when life is fraught with challenges. Chi Kung approaches recovery with the opposite priorities and emphasis: emotional self-regulation and relaxing the body are viewed as the necessary foundational pieces for people to then be able to think objectively and act, without emotions holding them back.

In the West, scientific research is highly valued as a guide to what treatment programs should include and what to emphasize in their offerings. In a sense, Chi Kung operates the same way. Research is certainly valued and has been used to shape and change Chi Kung practices for millennia. The difference is that Chi Kung has primarily relied on the systematic gathering and application of the experiences of its practitioners in natural settings. The practices were first developed by noting what adults, children, and animals do that help them feel better. Both approaches have their value. Modern research methods can isolate the effects of a treatment to assess its potency and staying power. Systematic observation over millennia has value in terms of testing approaches in the real world and everyday life over a

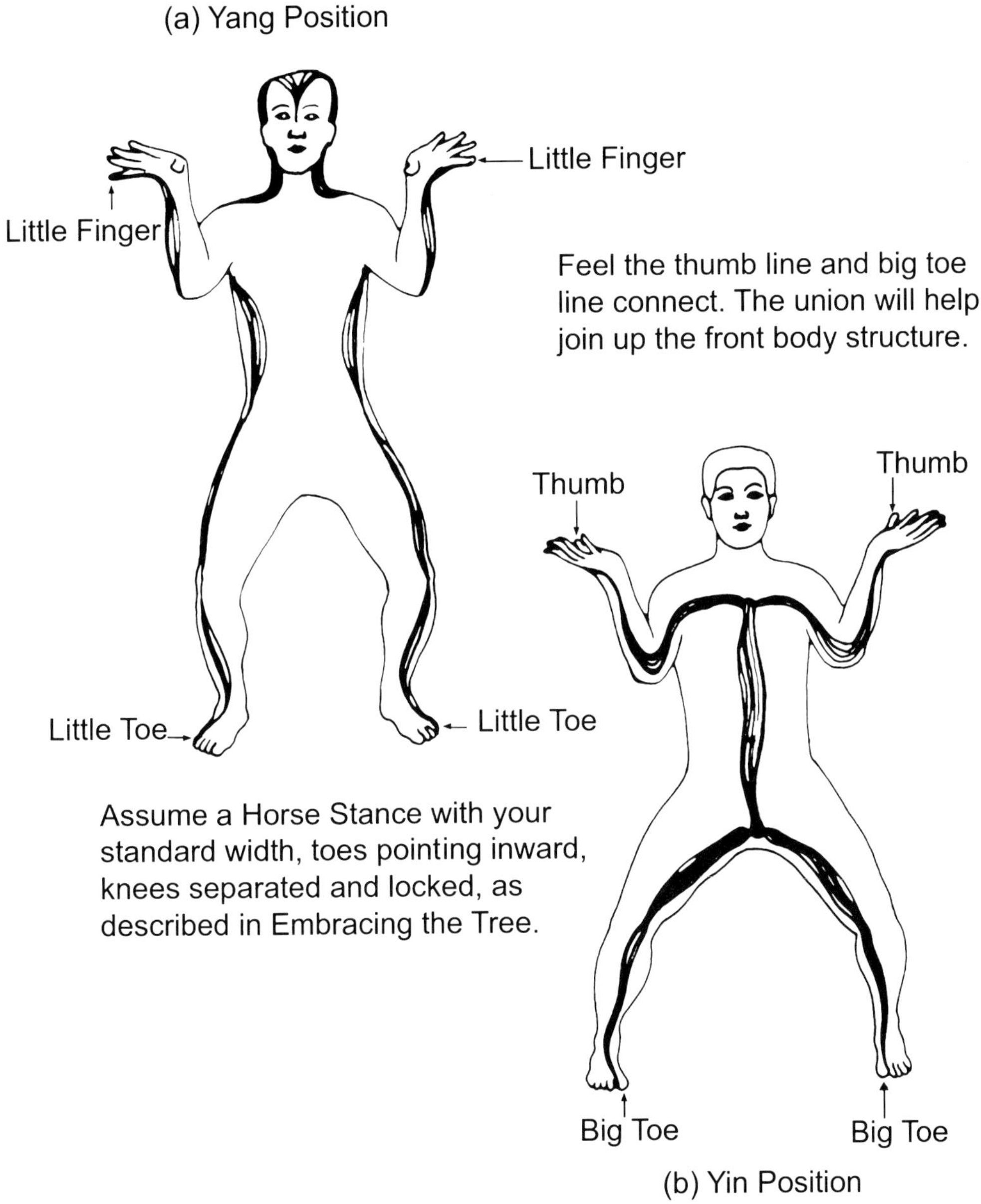

Fig. 3.2. An example of Chi Kung: Iron Shirt Chi Kung: Holding the Golden Urn

much larger expanse of time—thousands of years, in fact. This means that in the Taoist approach there are fewer expectations in terms of policies, procedures, and paperwork.

Naturally, since addiction treatment programs want to be effective and marketable, the emphasis is on results. Chi Kung does not ignore results, but it does not claim to "treat" anything. The intention instead is to teach people the practices that can heal them from the inside out and encourage them to practice regularly. The focus is more on process than achieving results. The effects of the practices and the path of healing for each person are individual. Programs based on the Western model of treatment tend to operate on the idea that the program is supposed to have at least some responsibility for "fixing" the person, and if the program cannot do that, then it is not a "good" program. In Chi Kung you are taught how to heal yourself, and the teachings are offered in a way that anyone can understand. It is then up to the person to practice. There is no way to predict how long the process will take or how many obstacles will be encountered along the way. Master Chia says, "You do it, you get it."

Western approaches to addiction treatment tend to start with the mind and only then consider the effects of the emotions on the body. Chi Kung works the other way around—from the body to the emotions to the mind. Both approaches have their value. Combining them in a treatment program creates a higher likelihood that all three levels will be positively affected by the treatment protocol. The Western approach that emphasizes using thinking to forge new habits through sheer willpower takes a lot of effort and diligence, and in the early stages of recovery this can feel insurmountable. Chi Kung, on the other hand, is often experienced as more enjoyable, even fun.

Detoxification from a Western perspective tends to be treated as a separate event from treatment, an initial event with a short duration that primarily involves removing toxic chemicals from the body. In Chi Kung, detoxification is an ongoing process that is part of the natural way the human body is designed to work. It involves purifying the body of all the toxins that we are often exposed to, whether they be environmental, emotional, or mental. It is believed that toxic emotions and thoughts, if unprocessed, will eventually become physical toxins.

Compared to the Western way of life, the Taoist approach to life might be considered countercultural. It encourages people to strive less, let go of attachments, and search for inner peace over material gain. Taoists would say that Chi Kung is not counterculture but simply a better culture. Recovery involves living in harmony with nature rather than struggling to conquer it, and that is viewed as being a healthier way of living. Western approaches to addiction recovery tend to value support from other people as an important part of a successful recovery. Chi Kung also values that kind of support, but it offers ways to draw support from the energy all around us as well.

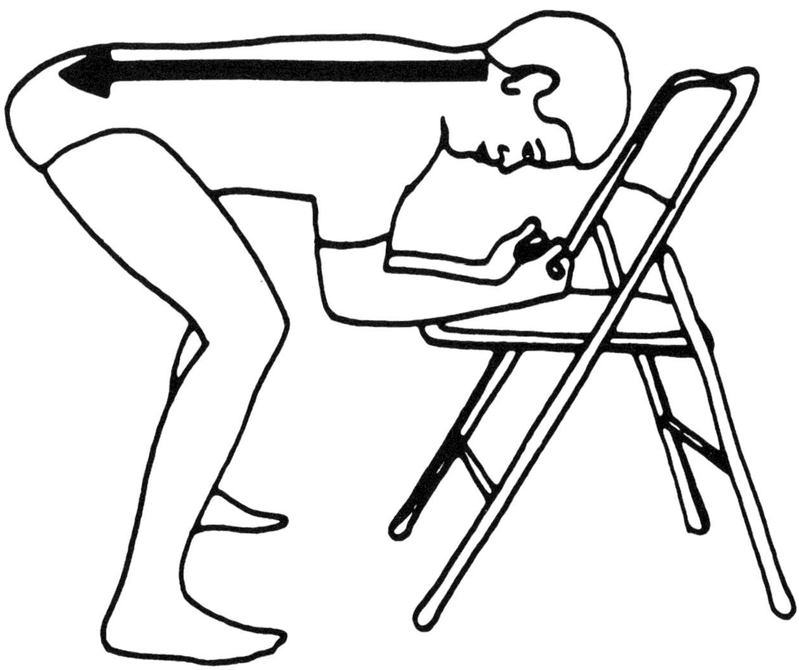

Fig. 3.3. An example of Chi Kung: Golden Turtle immersing in water and buffalo emerging from the water Chi Kung postures.

The role models in Western society tend to be people. All people have flaws, and so they can let us down when we need their help. "Do not meet your heroes," it is said. Chi Kung practices emulate nature, especially the wind and water. Water, for example, cannot be destroyed. It changes to adapt to its environment. Water, therefore, is a reliable role model. Some Western approaches to addiction treatment focus on eliminating the negative traits and situations that could stop people from stabilizing their recovery. Others focus on building on the positive qualities and situations that could benefit them. Chi Kung focuses on creating a balance between the negative and the positive, or on transforming the negative into the positive.

The Western approach involves diagnosing the negative and then trying to develop a strategy to address it based on the diagnosis. Chi Kung just teaches people how to be healthy and happy. The approach of many addiction treatment programs in the West focuses on addressing the individual parts of the problems that people have and trying to address those parts one by one. Chi Kung is focused on the whole, which includes the interaction of all the parts that comprise the whole.

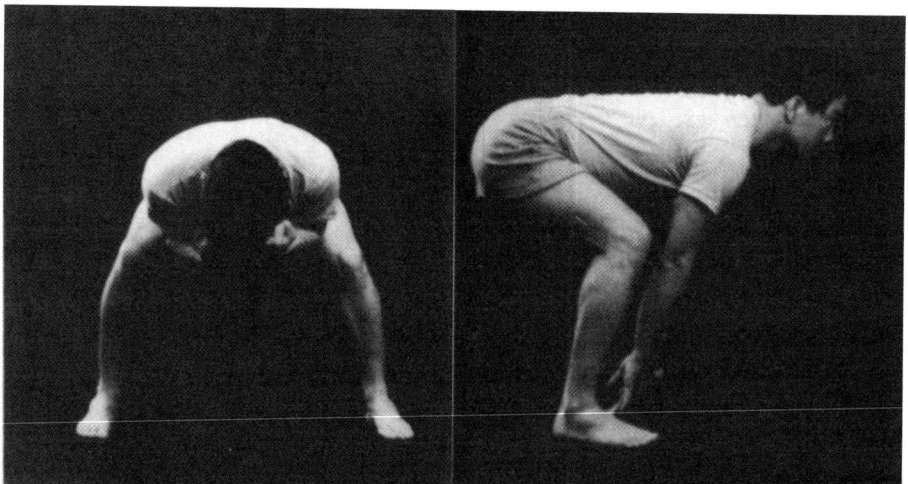

Fig. 3.4. An example of Chi Kung: Golden Phoenix washing its feathers Chi Kung postures.

Thus the Chi Kung view says that our internal organs comprise a complete and interrelated system, such that a problem in one organ will affect the others.

Chi Kung directly addresses issues that are often not addressed or not addressed sufficiently in most treatment programs. Examples of such issues would be how to increase compassion, get better sleep, improve your daily energy level, reduce or remove urges, shut off your brain, and address excesses or deficits of sexual energy. Many people in early recovery complain that they cannot concentrate enough to meditate. But when they try Chi Kung, they often find that the steps involved in each practice keeps their minds focused, so it's easier for them to meditate.

The Taoist approach to addiction treatment embraces anything that works. It seems reasonable that when it comes to any kind of chronic condition it is usually advisable to address the issue in as many ways as possible, as it is impossible to predict what will have the most beneficial impact for an individual. It might be something that someone said in a 12-Step meeting or a group session. It might be a particular piece of the healing process. It might be an impactful suggestion that is offered. In short, the idea behind the Taoist approach is to incorporate whatever works while integrating the appropriate Chi Kung practices so that the treatment program will have maximum benefit.

ANCIENT TAOIST KNOWLEDGE APPLIED

Taoism can help people understand how they can put certain important concepts in recovery into action in their lives. Rather than just thinking that they "should" do something that is generally viewed as being helpful for recovery, it is better if people can understand exactly how that approach fits in terms of living in harmony with nature and their surroundings. For example, moving away from the demands of the ego to a more humble stance is a standard recommendation in recovery. It is also a goal of Taoism. But why should you do that, though? There are plenty of examples of high-profile people who flaunt their abilities or accomplishments and seem to get away with it. The ancient foundational text of Taoism, the Tao Te Ching, provides insights and guidance. The following extracts are from Mantak Chia and Tao Huang's interpretation of this classic text as presented in their book *The Secret Teachings of the Tao Te Ching*:

Chapter 22

1. Those who boast of themselves lose their stance.
   He who displays himself is not seen.
   He who justifies himself is not understood. He who lashes out does not succeed.
   He who builds himself up does not endure.
2. In the sense of Tao,
   This is said to be eating too much and acting too much. It results in disgust.
3. Those who desire will not endure.

Further instructions extol the benefits of keeping the ego in check:

Chapter 56

1. Those who know, do not say.
   Those who say, do not know.
2. Close the mouth.
   Shut the door.
   Merge into light.
   As ordinary as dust.
   Blunt the sharpness.
   Unravel the entanglements.
3. This is called mysterious sameness.

4. You are not intimate by acquiring it.
   You are not distant in not acquiring it.
   You do not profit by acquiring it.
   You do not lose it by not acquiring it.
   You are not ennobled by not acquiring it.
   You are not disgraced by not acquiring it.
5. This enables the nobility of the world.

Overcoming perfectionism and striving are common hurdles for people in recovery. Taoism refers to a concept called nonaction. This doesn't mean doing nothing, but rather it means going with the flow of life rather than pushing against it. Consider the following:

Chapter 63

1. Do nondoing.
   Engage in non-affairs. Savor non-flavor.
2. Large or small, many or few, reward or punishment, are all being done through Action.
3. Seek what is difficult with ease.
   Effect what is great while it is small.
4. The most difficult things in the world are done while they are easy.
   The greatest things in the world are done while they are small.
5. The sage never plans to do a great thing.
   Thus, he accomplishes what is great.
6. Facile promises necessarily result in little trust.
   What is easy necessarily entails difficulty.
7. Thus the sage, through extreme trials, encounters no difficulty.

And:

Chapter 64

1. It is easy to sustain what is at rest.
   It is easy to plan for that of which there is not even a sign.
   What is fragile is easily broken.
   What is minute is easily dispersed.
2. Act upon it before it exists.
   Regulate it before it becomes chaos.
3. A massive tree grows from a little sprout.
   A nine-story building rises from a clod of earth.
   A thousand fathoms begin with a single step.
4. Those who impose action upon it will fail.
   Those who cling to it lose it.
5. So the sage, through nonaction, does not fail.
   Not clinging, he does not lose.
6. The common people's engagement in affairs fail prior to success.
7. So the saying goes, "Give as much careful attention to the end as to the beginning; then the affairs will not fail."
8. It is on that account that the sage desires not to desire and does not value goods that are hard to get.
   He learns not to learn and restores the common people's losses.
   He is able to support the nature of all things and, not by daring, to impose action.

Learning to let go of expectations and resentments about what one should own or be able to accomplish in life is important for peace of mind and spirit in recovery, as reflected in the AA adage "Easy Does It." Learning about the value of living a life that is less full of extreme highs and lows is important to reach that peaceful state.

Chapter 23

1. Yield, and retain integrity.
   In the depths of whirling, there is stillness.
   The hollow enables the plentiful.
   The old gives way to the new.
   The small allows for increase.
   Excess breeds confusion.
2. Therefore the sage holds oneself as the shepherd of the world.
3. He who does not display himself is seen.
   He who does not justify himself is understood.
   He who does not lash out succeeds.
   He who does not build himself up endures.
4. Therefore,
   Only the spirit of noncompetition makes things noncompetitive.
5. So the old saying, "yield, and retain integrity," is but a few words.

But when rightly understood, integrity returns.

Many people in recovery have historical issues with authority figures and are rebellious and reactive as a result. Those tendencies can create problems if the person does not find a way to change this pattern. Rather than focus on people to provide heroic or exemplary models of how to operate in life, Taoism takes another approach:

Chapter 80

1. Nothing in the world is softer and more supple than water.
   When confronting strength and hardness nothing can overcome it.
2. Using nothingness simplifies.
   Using water overcomes hardness.
   Using weakness overcomes strength.

There is no one in the world who does not know it, but no one can apply it.

3. So it is a saying of sages that:
   Whoever can bear the misfortune of the world is the ruler of the world.
4. Truthful speech seems paradoxical.

Taoism values the paradoxical and underrated power of being small. Understanding its power can help people find ways to stop trying to prove themselves to others. This in turn can help prevent someone from resorting to an addictive substance or behavior to medicate their frustration and disappointment when they feel unappreciated by the people around them.

Chapter 66

1. The reason why rivers and seas have the capacity for kingship over all the valleys is that they excel in low lines.
   That is why they have the capacity for kingship over all valleys.
2. Thus, since the sage wants to elevate the people, his speech is down-to-earth.
   Since the sage wants to advance the people, he positions himself at the back,
3. So that when he is at the front, people do not harm him.
   When he stands above, people do not feel pressure.
   The whole world supports him untiringly.
4. Since he does not rely on competition, the world has nothing with which to compete.

Understanding our personal strengths as well as our challenges of character is an important aspect of recovery. So is knowing what to do with them. People often become frustrated by trying to overcome

INNER TRADITIONS
BEAR & COMPANY

Affix
Postage
Stamp
Here

Inner Traditions • Bear & Company
P.O. Box 388
Rochester, VT 05767-0388
U.S.A.

tendencies that could lead them back into active addiction. Some of these tendencies may be part of an individual's personality, while others may have been present for so long that it's difficult to recognize or change them. Taoism offers another approach, one of acceptance and cooperation:

Chapter 2

1. In the world,
   Everyone recognizes beauty as beauty,
   Since the ugly is also there.
   Everyone recognizes goodness as goodness,
   Since evil is also there.
2. Since being and nonbeing give birth to each other,
   Difficulty and ease complete each other,
   Long and short measure each other,
   High and low overflow into each other,
   Voice and sound harmonize with each other,
   And before and after follow each other.
3. Therefore the sage
   Lives in actionless engagement,
   And preaches wordless doctrine.
4. The myriad creatures
   Act without beginning,
   Nourish without possessing,
   Accomplish without claiming credit.
5. It is accomplishment without claiming credit that makes the outcome self-sustaining.

On the surface, recovery seems simple. "Just stop using," some people might say. "Get ahold of yourself." "Get your priorities straight." It would be wonderful if it were that simple, but it isn't. If it were, people would do it. No one wants to have a life full of the chaos, drama, and pain that goes with addiction. People who are struggling to stabilize their recovery soon realize that under the surface there are many seeming paradoxes to the process of recovery. They have to slow down to speed up their recovery and let go to get control. These seeming contradictions are hard to understand and often even more difficult to put into practice. Taoism has been grappling with the wisdom of this conundrum for thousands of years:

> **Chapter 36**
>
> 1. When you want to constrict something,
> You must first let it expand;
> When you want to weaken something,
> You must first enable it;
> When you want to eliminate something,
> You must first allow it;
> When you want to conquer something,
> You must first let it be.
> This is called the Fine Light.
> 2. The weak overcomes the strong.
> Fish cannot live away from the source.
> The sharp weapon of the nation should never be displayed.

INCORPORATING THE TAOIST APPROACH IN TREATMENT

How can Taoist principles and Chi Kung practices be integrated into existing treatment programs? Questions arise about what aspects of such an integrated approach should be given priority, how much time should be devoted to each aspect, how individual needs can be taken into account without diluting the effectiveness of the program or losing the sense of connectedness between program participants, or how to avoid creating something that just seems like a hodgepodge of activities.

There are some fundamental ideas from Taoism that suggest how to successfully integrate Chi Kung practices in a recovery setting. We will borrow a term that is used in EMDR (Eye Movement Desensitization and Reprocessing) training: *creating space*. Imagine that your upper torso, from your waist to your neck, is where you store emotions about issues that are not within your control or understanding. In common discourse we often refer to shoving something under the rug to ignore it, and it seems that we tend to shove them down into our upper torso. Another common expression that seems to reflect an awareness of problematic issues taking up space inside of us is in the declaration, "I've had it up to *here* with [fill in the blank]." We seem to intuit that we stuff our unprocessed emotions somewhere in our bodies, that they take up space, and that eventually we run out of room for all those unprocessed feelings. We also seem to feel the weight of those unprocessed emotions. People say things like "I was crushed," "I was floored," and "It was too much weight for me to bear."

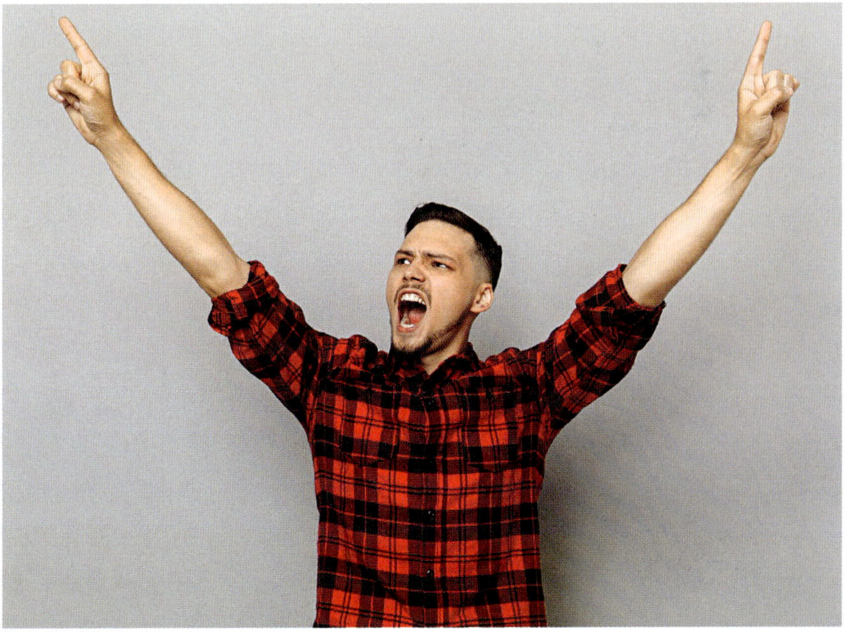

Fig. 3.5. I have had it up to here!

It's important that people who have addictions clear out as many of their unprocessed emotions as possible so that they will have room to deal with whatever comes next in their lives. Treatment programs need to make this a priority if they want their clients to have a fighting chance at staying clean and sober. The issues that they have not been able to let go of on their own need to be addressed as completely as possible in treatment. If they are not addressed, it would be too easy to blame someone for slipping by suggesting that they faltered because they did not put enough effort into treatment or because they are somehow too weak or not ready to stay on track. However, as long as those deeply buried issues are operating inside of us they will inevitably be triggered by something or someone; those afflicted with addictions will then find it very hard not to self-medicate.

The most meaningful issues are usually the ones that take up the most space. People sometimes chastise themselves (or others) for being so affected by a seemingly minor issue and assume that only issues that are conventionally associated with trauma, like being sexually assaulted or experiencing the horrors of war, need to be addressed with specialized approaches. That is not true. If someone is hurt by a person who means very little to them, it is usually easier to let go of any hurt feelings. However, if that person is someone who matters a great deal to them it's more likely that those hurt feelings will go unacknowledged and get stuck inside the person. In other words, it's not the size of the event that dictates how traumatic it will be for a person—it's how important that event is to the person who experienced it.

Let's consider again the idea of cumulative trauma. When someone searches their past for the source of their trauma they often limit their search to a significant single event. Examples are sexual, physical, or emotional abuse; car accidents; war experiences; or a devastating natural event. However, the accumulated emotional weight of smaller events that the person cannot understand or change for the better carries the same emotional weight as a single big event. Examples would be continual dysfunctional family dynamics or unresolved issues causing couples to argue and fight over and over again, never reaching resolution. As well, keep in mind that the loved ones of someone with an addiction are often overwhelmed with fear, worry, and the frustration of dealing with the addict's behavior over the time it takes before they go for help. Think of the accumulation of emotions as being like grains of sand piling up in an hourglass. If enough grains pile up, the person will eventually "flip."

Triggering memories can take up a lot of energetic space and increase the chances that the person will return to their addiction if they are not addressed. Moreover, people struggling with addictions paradoxically often had positive early experiences with what they're addicted to, in the sense that those experiences brought a kind of temporary relief. For example, the first high or the first taste of alcohol may have been an exhilarating experience that made them forget their pain. These early memories still tug at them, tempting them to revive that initial positive experience. Of course, at the same time they will also have shameful memories associated with their addiction that will cause them to want to further medicate those feelings. These kinds of triggers need to be addressed and neutralized, or the person will have to battle these unconscious urges using sheer willpower, which is always a losing battle.

Again, the frequent concern of administrators who run treatment programs is that addressing underlying trauma and its triggers will take up too much time. However, Chi Kung practices offer a way to address these emotional triggers through what is known as Taoist Emotional Recycling (TER), a practice found in chapter 10). When the emotions that take up too much space have been neutralized, the fight-or-flight mechanisms that cause a person to react are finally turned off. Once that happens, they are in a far better position to absorb, retain, and make use of the other useful tools that are offered in treatment. The foundational practices of the Universal Healing Tao system, such as the

Inner Smile (chapter 8), the Microcosmic Orbit (chapter 8), and the Six Healing Sounds (chapter 9), can help a person address unresolved feelings safely. These basic practices are good preparation for the TER practices found in the last chapter. If the person is feeling overstimulated by doing the foundational practices, they should just keep practicing them until they feel their emotions are manageable. At that point it will be safe to start TER.

Another suggestion focuses on the value of offering modules of treatment experiences as opposed to a single "one size fits all" approach in which everyone experiences the same protocol in a specific order. Modules are information and treatment sessions about a single topic that range from one hour to a few days in duration. Examples of topics for a module might be grief and loss, letting go, communication skills, and anger management. This kind of approach accommodates individual preferences and levels of readiness in treatment. The idea is that more than one module can be offered, and each module could be offered more than once in a treatment period. This way, participants can choose not only which issues they want to address, but the order in which they want to address them.

As we can all imagine, people come to addiction treatment facilities at varying levels of readiness and with different challenges. Some participants have attended programs before, so they are no doubt hoping for a new or different experience. Although it is not advisable to let people completely "run their own program," as it is referred to in the 12-Step community, it is also important to acknowledge that it will likely be easier for people to be motivated to learn and practice what they learn if they have some control over the sequencing of their treatment issues. It would also help them to mentally break their treatment experience down into manageable chunks. Accomplishing this could be as simple as including the following kinds of questions on an intake form and then providing a schedule of the modules that will meet each person's individual needs.

Sample Intake Questions

Do you want to:

1.	Learn to relax?	yes	no
2.	Learn to concentrate?	yes	no
3.	Learn about addictions?	yes	no
4.	Learn about recovery?	yes	no
5.	Learn about relapse prevention?	yes	no
6.	Learn couple skills?	yes	no
7.	Learn about codependency?	yes	no
8.	Learn how to reduce urges?	yes	no
9.	Learn how to get better sleep?	yes	no
10.	Learn how to improve self-esteem?	yes	no
11.	Learn about family dynamics?	yes	no
12.	Learn how to let go of emotions?	yes	no
13.	Learn how to balance your mood?	yes	no
14.	Learn how to have a healthy diet?	yes	no
15.	Clean out more toxins?	yes	no
16.	Understand yourself better?	yes	no
17.	Learn more about your beliefs?	yes	no
18.	Learn how to regulate sexual urges?	yes	no

Ideally, the client would have a check-in with the intake person at regular intervals throughout their treatment to see if their needs have changed. Inappropriate behavior or unwillingness to participate would also affect their treatment path.

The intake process itself could be expanded in other ways that add to the quality of the treatment experience. For example, if a program integrates energy work in its format, then the intake process should reflect that. Assessments at intake often include screening for suicide, homicide, clinical depression, anxiety, trauma, and other psychiatric conditions. They also find out which medications

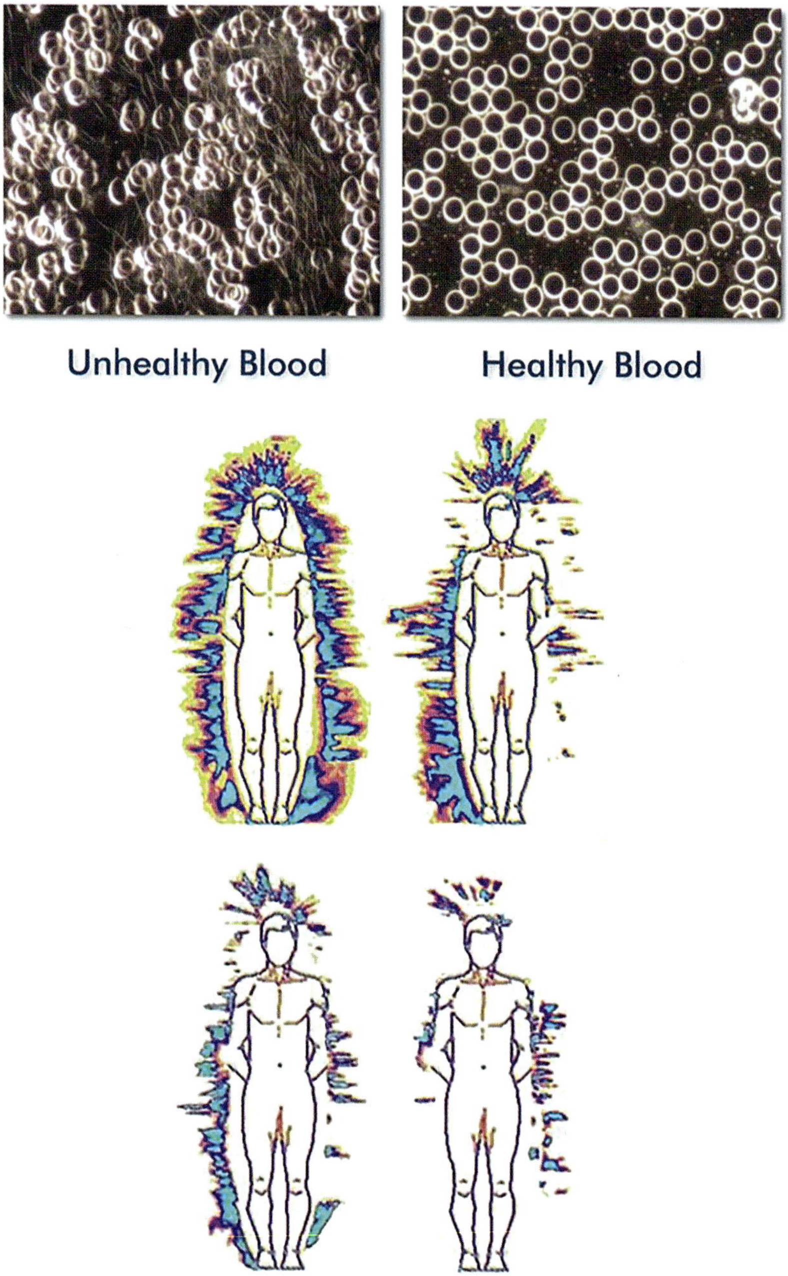

Fig. 3.6. Getting a more complete picture through holistic tools such as blood work and the Biopulsar Reflexograph.

participants are taking and what other treatment programs they may have attended. Urine testing for illicit substances is common in these programs. A more holistic approach could include such technologies as the Biopulsar Reflexograph, a biofeedback tool that gives scientific information and objective interpretations of the body's electromagnetic field and the seven major energy centers, or chakras; aura imaging; live blood (dark field) analysis; sugar and fats screening; bioterrain testing (urine, saliva, and physical testing); and breath analysis. In addition, to address the energetic issues that are identified in the assessment, programs could benefit from offering specific treatments such as colon hydrotherapy, far infrared sauna, lymphatic drainage, liver flush, and Thai massage, as well as Chi Nei Tsang, Karsai Nei Tsang, and Tok Sen practices.

Ongoing assessments should be done in any treatment program to make sure it is providing services that are in line with the intention of the

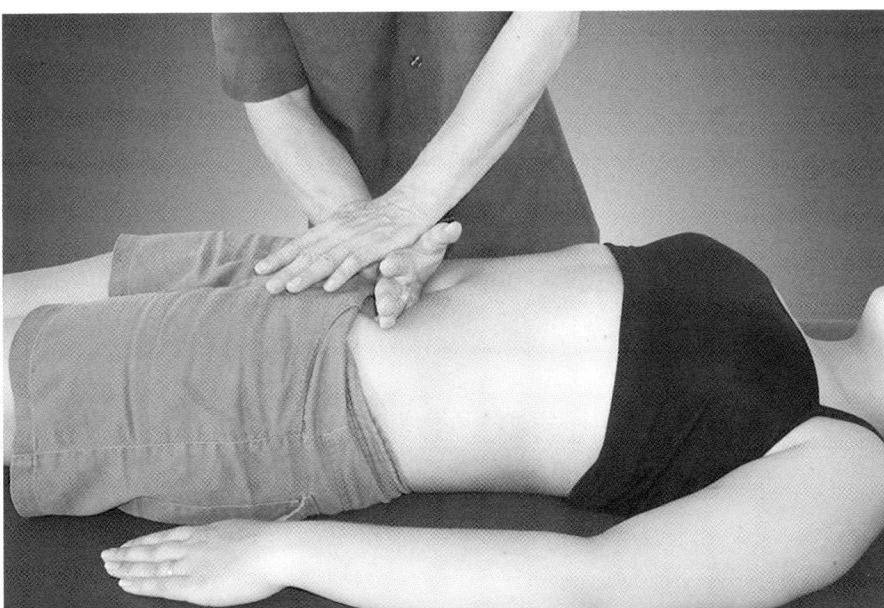

Fig. 3.7. Clean, balance, and strengthen your internal organs through Chi Nei Tsang treatment.

program and to assess the quality of service and the satisfaction of clients and staff. Open questions could be framed as:

- What have you learned?
- How has it helped you?
- What progress have you noticed that you have made?
- What parts did you like best?
- What parts did you like least?
- What would you add or change to make the program better for you?

4

Yin and Yang and the Concept of Balance

To understand how the practices offered later in this book can help someone purify, balance, and strengthen their energy, it is useful to more closely examine the concepts of yin and yang and how they interact.

The yin/yang symbol is familiar to most of us. We intuitively recognize it as the universal symbol of balance and harmony. It represents many important concepts in Taoism. The symbol has two joined halves, one white and one black. These two halves point to our dualistic perception of nature. We make comparisons in order to understand life around us. We unconsciously perceive the world around us in black and white, or we try to reduce it to that level to decide how to respond to any given life situation. For instance, when meeting someone new, most people usually try to assess whether that person is "good" or "bad." Yin energy (the black side) receives, gathers, nurtures, and stores. Yang energy (the white side) expands, exerts, and pursues. This can also be understood in terms of the negative and positive charges of a battery. They are also associated with masculine and feminine energies. Sometimes they are used to illustrate how conscious and unconscious aspects of people are different and connected.

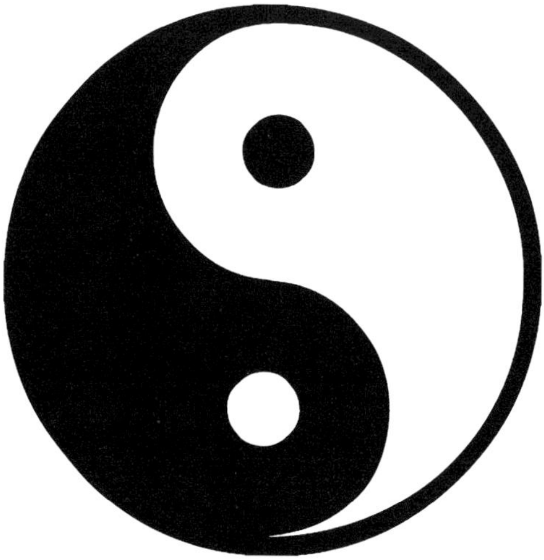

Fig. 4.1. The yin/yang symbol illustrates the power of opposites in balance.

Notice that the two halves of the yin/yang symbol are linked, and that their fishlike shapes complement each other to form a circle. This reminds us that we need both aspects for life to occur, that there is an upside and a downside to everything, that these opposing forces are part of a larger whole indicated by the circle, and that they interact with and influence each other. The circle indicates the ever-changing cycle of life—just looking at the symbol brings the idea of motion to mind. It is easy to imagine it rolling like a wheel. That notion can help people to accept the ups and downs of life and to focus more on trying to create peace and balance between the two sides rather than trying to get rid of the downsides. This can help people figure out how to avoid or get out of power struggles with the contradictory aspects of themselves, other people, or situations.

DUALITY AND ONENESS

Sometimes people think along the following lines: "I am right. I should get my way. Therefore, you should do it my way. If you don't do it my way, I should try to make you do it my way." This kind of thinking sounds aggressive when spelled out like this, but when these kinds of thoughts are unconscious, they can drive some rather extreme behavior. The yin/yang symbol can help people remember that there is another way to perceive that goes something like this: "I have my way, and you have your way. How can we get our two ways to work together so that we can both feel satisfied with the result?" Feelings are the bottom line for deciding whether or not the issue has been resolved. If one person gets their way and the other person is resentful, then the issue is not resolved, and it will probably come up again at some point. Many situations arising among people resist linear, logical solutions because they are cyclical problems. The diverging viewpoints may clash. As a result, people become more extreme in their responses, clinging ever harder to their viewpoints, leaving the impression that each side is overly controlling and does not care that much about the other side's viewpoint.

A simple example of this is when one partner in a couple relationship complains that the other partner does not do enough of the housework, and the other partner argues that the real issue is how much complaining the other partner does about it. They could argue endlessly if they take the logical, rational approach to solving the argument. The more one of them makes his or her point, the more the other will argue against it. They both have reason to be unhappy with the situation. They will sort it out quicker and with more satisfaction if they try to create a solution that is satisfactory for both of them. For example, they could agree to do the housework together and then do something they both enjoy afterward.

An example that is more directly related to addiction could be when worried loved ones try to tell someone that she or he has an addiction and needs to go for help to address it. The family and friends of the person with the problem often end up feeling frustrated by the response to their pleas. The more they argue for what they believe is right, the more the person they are confronting clings to their viewpoint. A better solution would be if the loved ones first made the person they are concerned about feel safe enough to talk about how they feel about overcoming their problem. Once the person realizes that their addiction is a problem and they decide to enter some sort of treatment program, they may subsequently feel hounded by their loved ones, who constantly monitor them, reminding them to stay on track. Their friends and family members are worried about them, and based on the person's past behavior they have trouble trusting that he or she will do the right things to stay clean and sober without their constant monitoring (see "Codependency," chapter 1). They may have the best of intentions, but the person who is dealing with an addiction can feel suffocated and insulted by this kind of behavior when they are trying their hardest to prove that they are trustworthy. It's easy for people in this kind of situation to get caught up in a power struggle by trying to make the other party see their point of view.

A more effective strategy in such a situation would be to have regular meetings where the person in treatment can update the loved one(s) on his or her progress and can answer questions, knowing that those questions will be restricted to their agreed-upon meetings. Another solution would be to make an agreement that both parties will have periodic check-ins, maybe by text or video, so that the person in treatment can demonstrate that her or his recovery is on track, which would allow the loved ones to praise and encourage the person instead of giving unneeded or unwanted advice or reminders.

People can have these kinds of push-pull power struggles within their own minds, too, especially if they tend to overanalyze. An example would be when someone tries to change who they intrinsically are. Say this person admires people who are more extroverted and would like to be more like them. They want to feel comfortable in social situations and even be energized by them. However, if the person is an introvert by nature, they will not be able to become an extrovert no matter how hard they try. Some aspects of our personality are pretty much set by the time we reach adulthood. It would be more helpful in such a situation to realize that there are pros and cons to both extroversion and introversion, that people have both tendencies to some extent, and that they can accept their personalities and capitalize on their strengths rather than envy people who have different personalities.

People who have addictions are often plagued by guilt and shame after they start recovery. They remember all the things they did to feed their addiction and the responsibilities they neglected while they were actively using. They can use positive affirmations to try to keep from feeling bad about themselves, but at best this only works while they are repeating those affirmations. The struggle to defeat guilt and shame can be exhausting. Family strife happens periodically, but internal struggles with oneself can follow you around all day long. A better way to resolve this kind of internal power struggle might be to appeal to the yin/yang symbol and remind oneself of the difference between one's authentic self—who they truly are—and their addictive behavior. Then they can more readily avoid self-blaming for things that happened when they were heavily involved in addiction.

It should also be noted that power struggles over which counseling approach is the best can also occur among the staff and contractors working in addition treatment facilities. Of course, a service provider has the right to make decisions about what kinds of services they offer. Individual counselors also have the right to decide what counseling approach suits them best, and most will believe in the efficaciousness of some approaches over others. In an attempt to promote their preferred approach as "the best," administrators may be tempted to force their counselors to adopt a particular approach. If it is not what the counselors already believe in or if it was not made explicit that that was the plan before they were hired, a power struggle usually ensues. Again, rather than trying to defeat each other it would be more effective if administrators and counselors focused on finding areas of agreement and capitalized on those to create a win-win situation.

BALANCING THE YIN ORGANS

People who have addictions often believe that they do not fit in with the rest of society. They see themselves as outsiders, as the "black sheep" of their families. They believe they think differently than the "normies" (a term used in 12-Step meetings that refers to people who do not have addictions) in their lives. Some of what formed their impressions of themselves came from judgments made by the people in their lives. If they grew up being called weird, bad, greedy, selfish, or any other pejorative, then they are more likely to believe that there is some truth to those comments. They also may have noticed that they do not think the same way as their friends and loved ones. That can lead them to think negatively about themselves instead of seeing the value in their uniqueness or viewing themselves as simply different instead of wrong or weird. They may have had negative experiences while trying to accept the generally accepted views of society, rejected those views as a result,

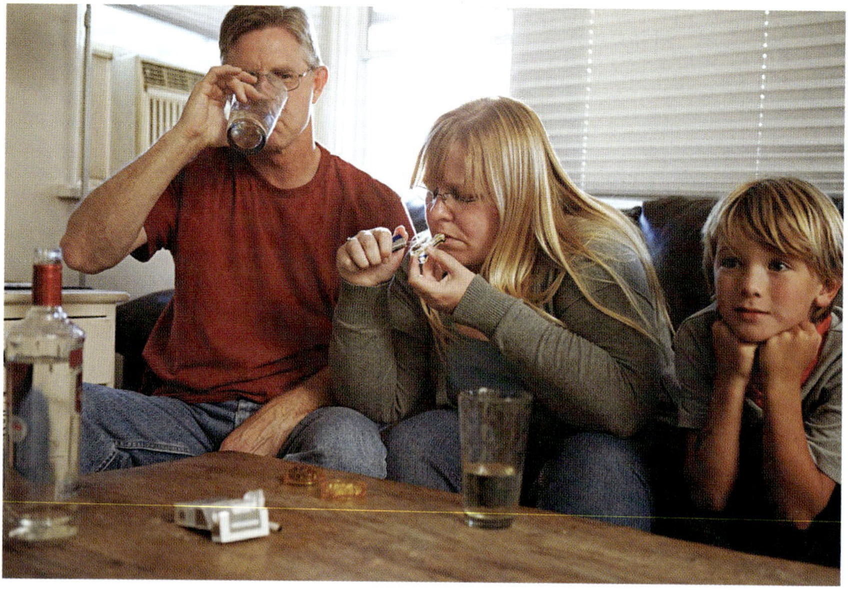

Fig. 4.2. Rejecting hypocrisy does not prevent people from acting in ways that they will regret.

and now define themselves in terms of being anti whatever the prevailing views are without necessarily knowing what they do believe in.

Children who have had negative experiences with church, for example, will reject religion without having a specific alternative to take its place. Viewing themselves as being on the fringes of society can lead them to find support and social contact with other people who have also rejected the ways of mainstream society. People who live with unprocessed resentment and shame are more vulnerable to becoming dependent on something addictive to medicate those feelings. At some point they may realize that in the process they have become someone who rejected people who advocated for a healthy lifestyle while living in unhealthy ways themselves. These realizations can reinforce the idea that they are not part of the mainstream, and this becomes a self-fulfilling prophecy.

Once someone starts using something addictive, the toxic effects of that substance start to accumulate in the body. If they carry negative feelings like shame or resentment over a long period of time, those emotions also condense to eventually become physical toxins. Physical and emotional toxins are like dust and dirt in your home, clogging up your energy channels and settling in your organs. When the yin organs are healthy and clean, they produce a specific set of virtues: The heart produces joy, happiness, and love. The spleen produces openness and trust. The lungs produce courage and righteousness. The kidneys produce calmness, gentleness, and stillness. The sexual organs produce creativity and vitality. The liver produces generosity and kindness. When these organs are healthy, clean, and strong, you will feel compassion (including compassion for yourself), have more optimism, and feel lighter inside. The virtuous and healthy chi in each organ helps the other organs in a creative cycle.

When these organs are negatively affected by toxins, what is produced are negative emotions and thoughts. The heart produces impatience, hastiness, and hatred. The spleen produces worry, negative

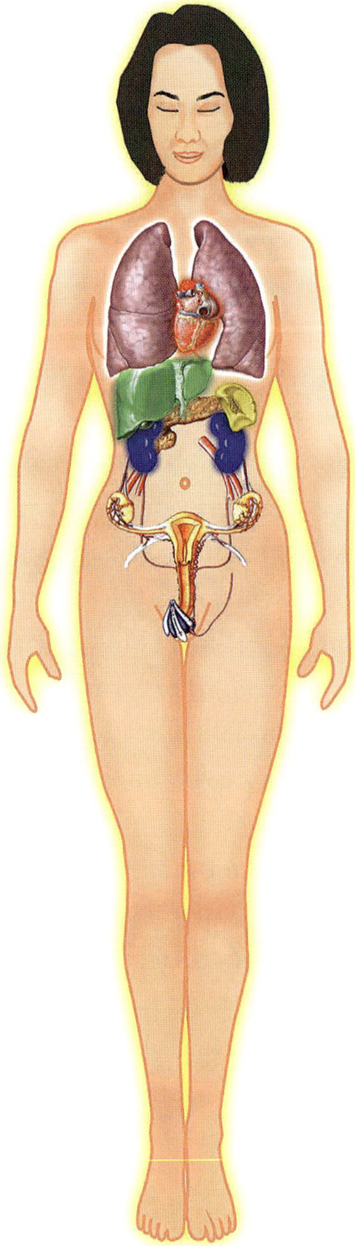

Fig. 4.3. Virtue is more than a mental state; it is also found in the organs.

thinking, and overthinking. The lungs produce grief, sadness, loss, and depression. The kidneys produce fear, stress, anxiety, and guilt. The sexual organs produce a lack of creativity and a lack of vitality. The liver produces anger, frustration, jealousy, envy, and resentment. Shame seems to come from all of them. The unbalanced and toxic energy in each organ not only weakens the specific organ, it weakens all the other organs in a destructive cycle.

The type of energy that is produced by each of the yin organs is different. The energies each function similarly to that of an element. The energy produced by the heart is warmer and more expansive, like fire, for example. Depending on the order in which the energies of the organs are activated and cultivated, they can either build on or destroy each other. Wood added to a fire can create more fire, for instance, whereas metal can chop wood. The order of activation also affects how the respective emotions of each organ affect each other. The order in

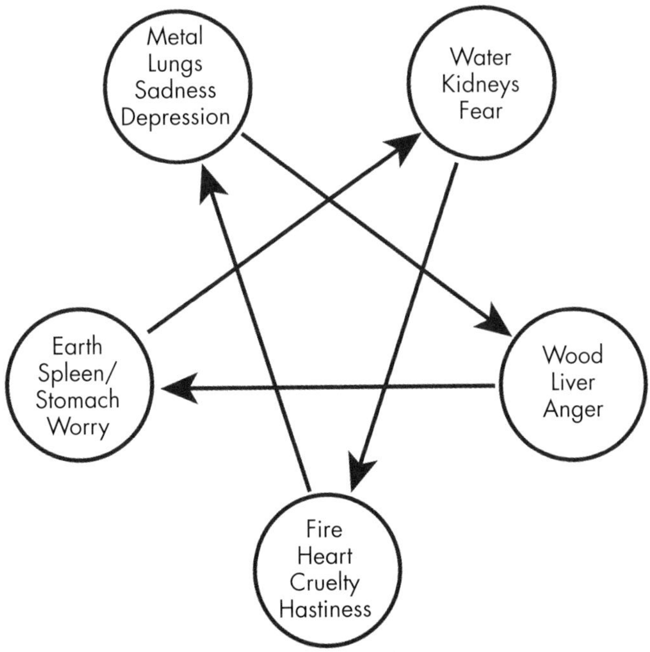

Fig. 4.4. Destructive cycle of the internal organs.

which one works with the organs can either strengthen or weaken the emotional processing system and either cultivate the virtues of each organ or bring forth their negative emotional states.

In chapter 8, we will discuss mood and organ health in greater detail, as well as learn the Inner Smile, a practice that helps to balance energy and transform vices into virtues.

When people who have addictions get into recovery, they soon learn that there are certain emotions, behaviors, and attitudes that appeared when their addiction first started and became stronger as their addiction progressed. These are called "character defects" in 12-Step parlance. They need to be recognized by the person in treatment so that they can change them, otherwise they might lead the person back to their addiction. Often people have difficulty managing those tendencies; they do not just fade away once the person enters recovery. Willpower, analysis, and self-monitoring have only a limited effect; when people try to simply make them go away, they often come back with a vengeance in some other way that they could not have anticipated. For instance, a man will try to forgive his father through sheer willpower and finds that his suppressed anger toward his father tends to explode if he gets triggered by someone who seems to repeat the original betrayal by his father.

Part of the reason these negative emotions, behaviors, and attitudes are so difficult to manage is because they do not originate in the mind. The negative effects of toxins on the yin organs comprise a fairly long list of "character defects." Learning how to balance, strengthen, and purify the chi in those organs through the practices of the Universal Healing Tao can provide people with practical and effective tools to transform those toxic effects into virtues.

Some people believe that they have an addictive personality. This implies that they are vulnerable to becoming addicted to many different things compared to other people, and they are usually active in more than one addiction at any given time. Their history of becoming dependent on several different addictive things tends to lead them to that conclusion. Sometimes that can also lead them to conclude that they are less likely to be able to maintain recovery or that the relapse prevention skills and strategies that work for most people will not work for them.

It is true that abstaining from one addiction could easily lead someone to switch to another, but that is true for almost everyone. A common example would be when someone stops smoking cigarettes and then starts eating more to cope with the craving to smoke. Another would be when people stop drinking and then throw themselves into their work to distract themselves from the desire to drink. People who have an addiction to something that strongly affects their dopamine levels—say, cocaine—can easily end up turning to another addiction that produces similar effects. The typical substitutes are gambling, carbohydrates, sex, the internet, and shopping. If the effects of an addiction on the internal organs are not properly addressed, the person will tend to automatically search for other addictive activities or substances that will produce similar effects.

THE MIRROR CONCEPT

Note that each of the two halves of the yin/yang symbol has a small dot of the opposite side inside it. The black side has a white dot and vice versa. Those dots convey the idea that nothing is completely good or bad in life. The dot reminds us that the addiction is only the person's behavior and not the true, authentic person. We all have that black or white dot. People who are dealing with addictions are not unlike anyone else.

Notice as well that each half of the symbol is widest where the other one comes to its narrowest point. This reminds us that when we sharpen and harden our beliefs and perspectives, we will eventually come closer to the other perspective. This usually comes as a surprise to people. Religious groups can end up operating from a place of vengeance, hatred, or judgment, even though their religion advocates for peace, love, and harmony. Someone who judges their family members who have a history of addiction may swear that they will never have an addiction but often end up with one anyway (although they often end up with a different addiction than the one their family members had). People remember how their parents treated them and vow to never act like that when they become parents, only to find themselves acting and speaking in similar ways when they become parents. A common saying is that there is a fine line between genius and madness. In the 12-Step program the fourth step advises participants to take an inventory of themselves, not of other people. This advice is directed at those who come to a meeting hoping not to be judged and to develop their own ideas about what works and what doesn't in recovery, but who later start to judge others by their own personal standards.

The yin/yang symbol encourages us to move beyond our black-and-white perceptions to find common ground or compromise. The symbol is never seen with just the white side or just the black side. This reminds us that we cannot destroy or ignore one side of the experience just because it does not appeal to us. It is important to understand and accept both sides. That is what's needed to reach a workable solution. A common saying is that once you completely understand the problem, the solution is obvious. Another common saying is that the solution to our problems often lies in the unappealing and the unexplored. The dots within the yin/yang symbol encourage us to suspend our judgments and explore the side that is less desirable or less familiar to us.

This kind of approach has important implications for how addictions are treated. Suppressing judgments of others or oneself can only last as long as the willpower of the person remains unbendable. Lasting resolution is more feasible if people get to know the payoffs of becoming familiar with their shadow side, the parts of themselves that are hard to face. Then they can figure out how to get those payoffs in healthier ways. In the 12-Step program, people often dread doing step four, the one where they're supposed to do an inventory of their character assets and defects. Naturally, the idea of spending a significant amount of time looking at the mistakes you've made and the flaws you perceive in your character is not something that you're excited about—it's a scary prospect. However, you might be more enthused about it if you approached step four with the intention of trying to figure out what needs you were trying to meet when you acted in ways that you now regret, and then figure out what healthy alternatives you can use to meet those needs in the future.

The yin/yang symbol can also be used to guide us to think about our struggles in more constructive ways. The question about why bad things happen to good people is one that no one can answer for sure. There are lots of theories, though. Some will say that it is God's will and that the Lord works in mysterious ways. Some will say we attract that which occurs in our lives, that our external world is influenced by what we focus on in our minds. Some believe it is the work of some shadow elite groups that control the direction of the world in secret. The yin/yang symbol can be used to help a person look at their circumstances as if they were a mirror image of their internal state. The black and white sides of the symbol are interlocked such that by turning them we see that the narrow part of one side is connected to the bulging side of the other, and vice versa. Similarly, your image is reversed when you see yourself in a mirror. Using the metaphor of a mirror, you can view your challenges and struggles as external reflections of your inner dialogue. Like a real mirror, the reflection is not exactly the original. Then you can examine your history and beliefs to look for patterns in those struggles and use that information to try to address not only your current circumstances, but the internal issues that might be connected to them or even fueling them. You cannot possibly know if that perspective is connected to any of the other possible explanations for why your life has turned out a certain way, but it at least provides a viewpoint that can lead you to constructive change over the things that are in your power to address. This approach reflects a different attitude about life—rather than viewing your situation as a threat with obstacles to be conquered, it is viewed as a reflection of your own inner imbalances, and you can use this insight to learn and grow.

For instance, a woman might wonder why she keeps meeting men who turn out to be jerks. She might therefore conclude that she is a magnet for jerks. So she watches more carefully for signs that the next man she meets is not a good person so that she can recognize and end her pattern, but this strategy doesn't quite work. There could be many reasons why she keeps finding herself in this kind of situation. Maybe it has something to do with where she goes to meet men. Maybe she is only attracted to men who treat her badly and she has forgotten about all the men she's met who treated her well. Maybe she likes men who have a bit of an edge or she favors bad-boy types. Maybe she does not feel comfortable with flirting and so the men who approach her are the ones who are bold enough to pursue her despite the absence of signals that she is even interested in them. These bold men might also be bold in undesirable ways. Maybe there were addictive substances or activities in the situation when she met those men and her judgment was impaired. Maybe she has unresolved trauma or abuse issues with a parent that she is unconsciously reenacting. Maybe she is just getting started with dating and has overgeneralized about all men based on a couple of bad experiences.

The reasons why someone might be dealing with this kind of issue are individual, of course, and there is often more than one factor involved if it is a pattern. This is where the mirror concept of the yin/yang symbol can be a helpful way to redirect the focus of the woman away from expectations, blame, self-pity, hopelessness, or a victim stance. The idea of the mirror suggests that the woman's pattern with men could be a reflection of other factors that need to be addressed; by perceiving this way, the woman can be encouraged to try to discover what this pattern reflects in herself so she can start looking at the true source of her problem rather than trying to pin it on some external source.

The Chi Kung practices that are offered in this book represent practical applications of the principle of yin and yang and the meanings of the yin/yang symbol. All the practices have the elements of both exertion (yang) and nurturing (yin). They all help anyone who practices them to connect with the pace and balance of nature. These practices are done with gentleness and patience, and so they teach us how to get in the habit of treating ourselves and others in that same way. The natural breathing technique that is used while performing the practices sends a message to the body that they can move out of a fight-or-flight crisis mode and can get used to living a life that is calm and peaceful and not filled with chaos and drama.

FINDING THE BALANCE IN LIFE

The practices of Chi Kung teach us how to balance yang energy with yin energy to restore and rejuvenate. They work with the energy channels or meridians that move through the body from each of the organs to distribute chi throughout the body. These practices are rooted in ancient knowledge and yet they are practical applications of the concepts that underlie quantum physics. Chi Kung practices reflect the idea that time and space may be how we register our reality through our senses, but we can look beyond these sensory inputs to draw the healing energy of chi into ourselves and further cultivate it. The practices work with the concept that despite what our senses tell us, we are all connected. The energy that fuels us is not just inside us, it's all around us, and we can influence and be influenced by that energy.

There are specific practices that are designed to maintain and restore health in areas that are often affected by addictive activities and are not often treated or are not treated completely when people go for professional help. Examples of such concerns: brain fog, tightness in the spine, pain in the joints, poor willpower, a lack of assertiveness, low self-esteem and lack of self-confidence, low energy, poor sleep, an inability

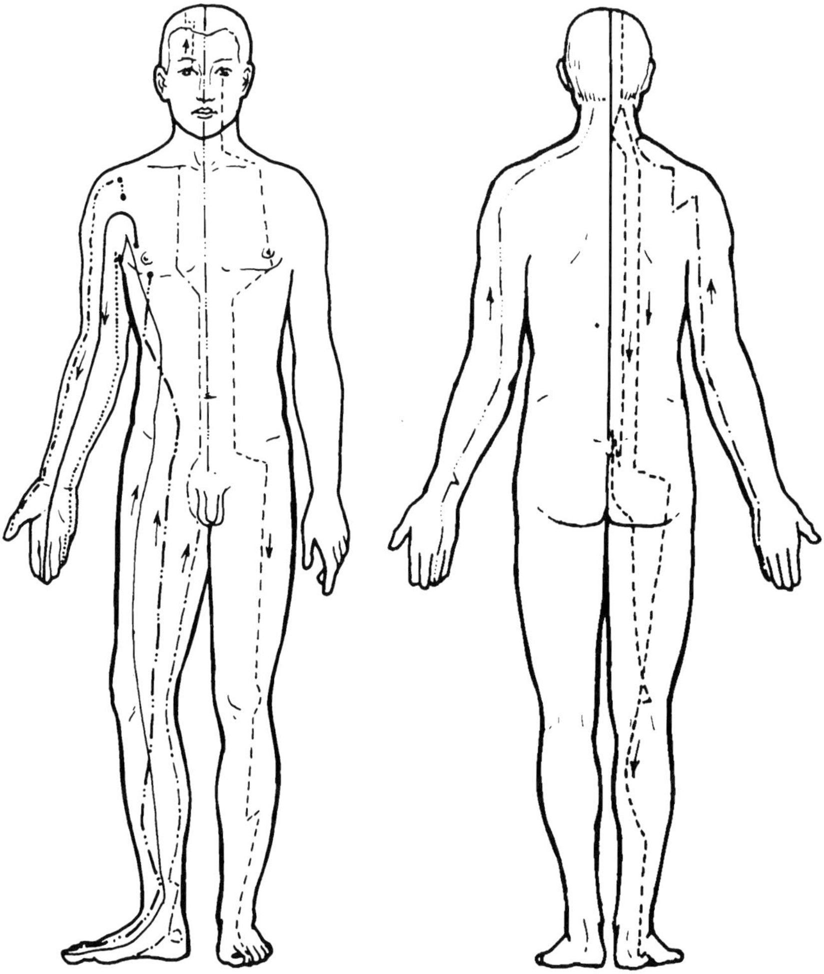

Fig. 4.5. The energetic river and streams of the human body.

to feel compassion, and too much or not enough of a sex drive. Specific practices will be described in this book for each of these concerns, many of which are classified as stage two concerns in addiction recovery. Stage one involves stopping one's involvement in the addictive activity or substance. Stage two has to do with what the person is going to do now they've stopped using to meet the needs that the addiction was initially trying to address, but in healthier ways. People often struggle with stage two because they have not had healthy hobbies or interests for a long time. The Universal Healing Tao system provides a wide selection of simple and effective practices that can allow anyone to learn how to be healthier and happier. It makes learning and practicing self-regulation fun and achievable.

By practicing the ancient methods of Taoism, we can learn how to feel lighter, stronger, happier, and more energetic. The practices show us how to create a sense of inner spaciousness and peace. The mood these practices foster provides a balance between high and low, which is something that people with addictions would ideally like to experience. That is the magic that we are all trying to achieve so that we have more control over how we feel. In truth, what we really want is not material possessions, but inner health and a sense of well-being. What good is having lots of money and possessions if you do not feel happy or well? Imagine how much we could positively impact the world with its crime rates, wars, and drug trade if we could teach people how to cultivate compassion and an inner sense of wellness and peace.

The Universal Healing Tao system teaches us how to transform negative energy into positive energy. That way we do not have to fear negative experiences. We can use that negative energy as raw material to create positive energy within ourselves in the same way that a lump of coal can be transformed into a diamond, or that a grain of sand inside an oyster can become a pearl. From the Taoist perspective, treatment is mostly about teaching people how to self-heal rather than trying to "fix" people who struggle with addictions. This type of approach can provide new ways to help people both in terms of prevention and treatment. It can also point the way toward a new culture that prioritizes internal over external gratification. Creating internal space is far more achievable than acquiring material space and does not create as much conflict in the process. Once people understand the concepts of yin and yang, the meridians, and their connections to the forces, elements, colors, sounds, and smells of nature, then they

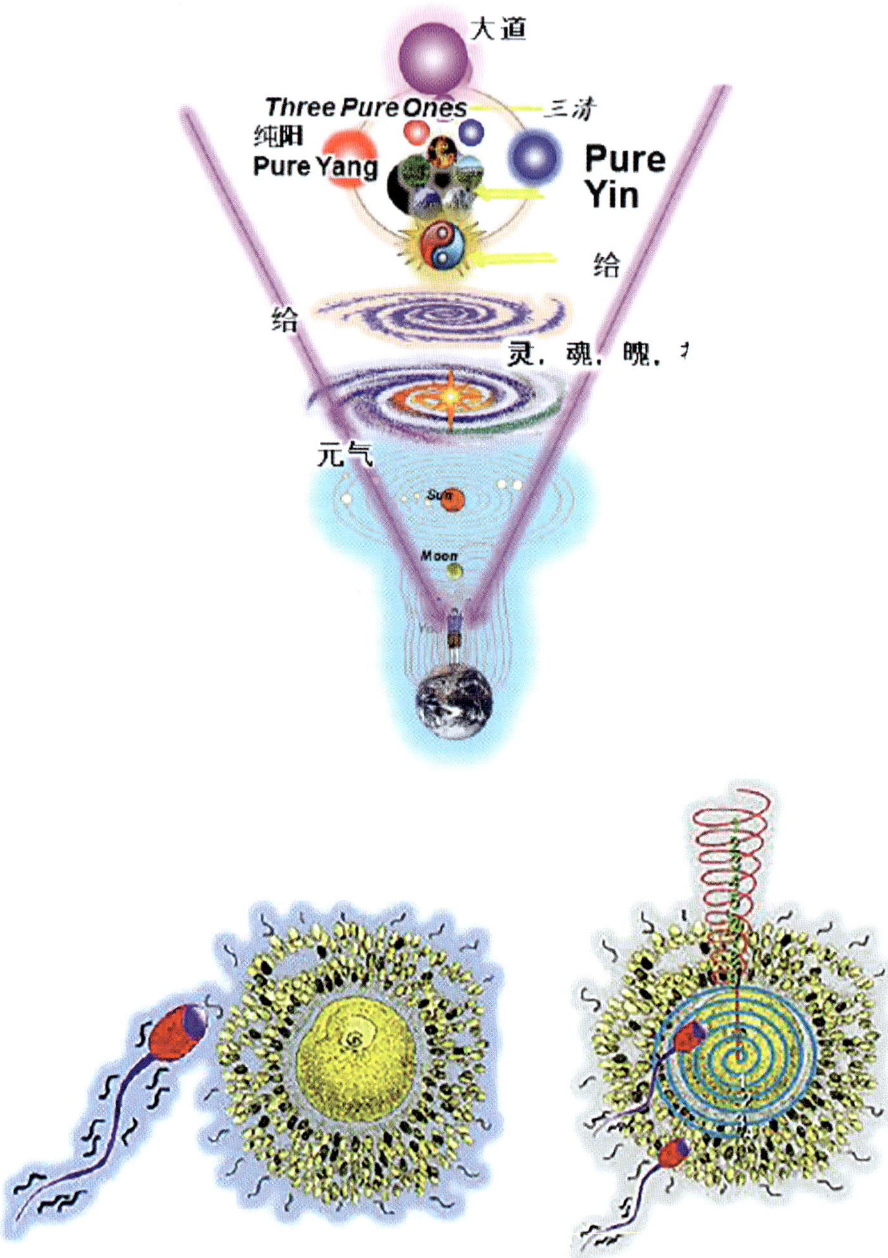

Fig. 4.6. Returning Home. Taoism encourages us to connect with nature and the universe so we can become light, clean, and whole—just as we were when we first entered this world.

can apply those concepts to create a sense of well-being and make healthy choices. This way of working with the natural forces of the universe goes beyond addiction treatment and can be applied to how one organizes one's home (feng shui), what food one chooses to eat, what clothing one chooses to wear, and how to make the most of one's personality tendencies.

The goal of learning the practices of the Universal Healing Tao system is to resolve the blocks that prevent us from becoming light, clean, and whole like we were when we first entered this world. One day we will each pass away and return to Source. The belief of the Universal Healing Tao is that we cannot accomplish this human journey if we are filled with toxins and negative emotions.

5

Getting Started with Chi Kung Practice

The different practices in this book have similar benefits: they all help us feel more relaxed, peaceful, energetic, and happy. Engaging in these practices on a regular basis provides concentration training, detoxification, and paths through which people can feel more connected internally and externally regardless of how enjoyable their social lives and family connections are. They allow people to experience and get comfortable with the yin side of life by slowing down, striving less, letting go, and appreciating a life of fewer extremes. They also provide both treatment and prevention benefits. Each of the practices has unique benefits, so it is best to practice all of them to get the full basketful of benefits. The practices do not have to be practiced all in one day or practiced every day. You can practice them at a pace that is manageable for you. Best of all, Chi Kung practices are not just for recovery from addiction or for those who are supporting someone in recovery; they will create a sense of well-being for anyone. Since this is the case, those who are trying to address their addictions need not feel burdened or ashamed about practicing them, as they are not practices specifically for someone with a problem—they are for everyone.

The basic Chi Kung practices in these chapters have been selected to address some of the most common challenges in recovery, and they are easy to learn. When you try them out, please keep certain ideas in mind:

First of all, be gentle with yourself. Being perfectionistic or setting high standards will not produce better results and certainly will not allow you to enjoy the experience to the fullest. Your ability to feel the benefits of these activities is likely to improve over the time you practice them, so there is no rush to master them. So be patient with yourself. Proceed slowly. Try not to practice when you are in a hurry or you feel very tired. Lower your expectations of what you think should happen when you practice. It works far better if you treat the experience of learning and practicing with curiosity and a playful attitude. If you expect to feel supercharged, like some kind of superhero, after you practice, you will be disappointed. But if you just wait to see what happens, you may be pleasantly surprised. Above all, do not strain or tighten up when doing the practices.

PRELIMINARIES

Before you begin, take some time to calm down and get grounded. Do not try to switch quickly from a hectic day to starting Chi Kung practice. Choose a place to practice that is quiet, peaceful, and feels safe. You do not have to do all of the practices in this book in a row or in rapid-fire succession. Think quality versus quantity. If you start to lose focus and become restless, then take a break or stop. You may have more satisfaction and better results if you sprinkle your practices throughout the day. See what works best for you, stay relaxed, and rest if you want to or need to.

Note that sometimes the practices that are the least appealing are actually the ones that you need the most. Practice them all. The way in which you approach the practices is also important. They are meant to be practiced slowly, gently, like water in a stream or a gentle breeze. Practice in such a manner that you feel calm. Notice that we commonly say "calm down," not "up." To calm down is to cool off. When we are not calm, heat and friction build up inside of us. Heat stops at the top of the body, at the head. This causes a lot of thoughts to whiz around inside of us, making it difficult to concentrate or think constructively. We tend to be more reactive because the fight-or-flight response is activated. Just remember, under stress we regress. This is literally true. When we are feeling overwhelmed, we are probably not eager to learn something new, even if it might work better. We are more likely to do what is more familiar to us, which we probably learned at a time when we were not as effective in life as we have become with more experience.

A concept that might remind you to avoid getting too stressed during your practice time involves what is known as state-dependent learning. It's a fairly simple concept that says that we tend to remember things when we are in the same state we were in when we first learned the information. We learn most of the best things there are to learn when we are calm, and we are more likely to remember them when we are in that state as well. Practicing while calm helps you connect that experience to all the other useful tools you learned while in that state. Then when life becomes difficult and you start to practice and become calmer, your stored wisdom will be more accessible, including your Chi Kung practices.

As well, develop a flexible practice routine. You could space out all of the practices in this book over a period of a week, for example. You could change which practices you do each day to prevent your routine from becoming stale. Then eventually you will not have to remember to practice or think too much about what practices to use each time. The routine will become automatic. You do not have to think too much to brush your hair or your teeth. You do those things every day. Eventually your Chi Kung routine will be the same. Then as soon as you start to calm down while practicing, you will remember why you practice and which practices to use that day.

To get the maximum benefit from the practices it's important to prepare properly. This includes repeating your commitment to stay away from your addiction, even if your commitment does not feel wholehearted yet. Make a list of the people, places, and situations that have or could trigger you to want to return to your addiction and remain committed to staying away from those triggers. The more you repeat those commitments, the more you will strengthen your resolve. Remember, triggers are not necessarily conscious or logical. If something in your life has been part of the routine that eventually led you to feed your addiction in the past, but it has no conscious or logical connection to your addiction, stay away from it anyway or change the routine. For example, many people have had the experience of unexpectedly encountering a certain smell that instantly brings them back to a memory from long ago. Triggers for addiction work the same way. Do not just ask yourself if thinking about or being near a certain trigger bothers you or makes you think about wanting to feed your addiction. That's not the issue. It is more important to ask if there is any chance that it might, even indirectly or over time, nudge you back toward your addiction. Then err on the side of caution. Remember, subtle triggers can be powerful because they do not seem dangerous enough to be taken seriously.

You may have to stop associating with certain people or places from your past even if they are near and dear to you, at least for a while. Make a list of quick and simple excuses or responses to the people you might run into who might try to persuade you to return to your addiction, so that you do not have to scramble for words in the moment. Remember, keep your responses short. "No" is a complete sentence. People who want to change your mind can twist your words around and try to use them to convince you. Be aware of that and remain resolved.

We know that when it comes to addiction, the old saying "Where there's a will there's a way" applies, but putting distance or obstacles between yourself and your addiction will help you to stay focused on your recovery. Stay away from things that could lower your inhibitions and return you to your addiction, like alcohol or marijuana, even if those substances are not your addiction. Limit your access to your specific addictive substance or activity as much as possible. Ideally you will have completely stopped using your addictive substance or activity for at least a few days before you start practicing.

Practicing Chi Kung is not likely to immediately override your desire to feed your addiction. Certainly the benefits of Chi Kung will not be noticeable or lasting if you keep using what you're addicted to—that would be like having a humidifier and a dehumidifier operating at the same time in the same room. Do whatever you can to clean out your system and detoxify before you start practicing. Drink plenty of water, eat plenty of leafy green vegetables, get some light exercise, have a sauna, go for acupuncture, get a massage, or maybe get some colonic treatments. Chi Nei Tsang, internal organ chi massage that quickly releases negative emotions, tensions, and sickness and brings comfort and relief to the abdomen and vital energy to the internal organs, it is a practice of the Universal Healing Tao that systematically detoxifies, balances, and strengthens the organs and their energy pathways throughout the body. There are practitioners all over the world. Maybe you can find someone in your area and get some treatments.

Make a list of the behaviors and attitudes that you have always had or have developed since you became addicted that could lead you back to your addiction. Then make a list of what you will practice instead to offset those tendencies. Be reasonable about what you can change and the time frame for change. Aim for small improvements and give yourself credit for each step you take in the direction of your goals. For example, some introverted people may wish they were more extroverted. They are aware that some of their desire to use addictive things stemmed from wanting to be more comfortable in social situations. It is impossible to completely change from an introvert to an extrovert, but such a person may be able to come up with strategies that can help in social situations, like breathing exercises, affirmations, and realizing that you can be interesting without being extroverted.

DEVELOP AN ATTITUDE OF GRATITUDE

Practice gratitude. A simple gratitude exercise is to think of three things that you are grateful for every day. Make sure you do not use items in your gratitude list that you can discount in some way. For example, "I am grateful for, but . . ." That "but" does not reflect gratitude. It ends up expressing resentment or disappointment. Practicing gratitude, even if you give thanks for the same three things in your list every day, helps to get your mind moving in a positive direction. You can start each item on your list with "I am grateful that/for . . ."

Some things to give thanks for might involve your home, community, family, friends, experiences, knowledge, health, possessions, country, improvements, or accomplishments. Give thanks to a Higher Power, however you define it. You may have already noticed that your mood has a momentum. When people start thinking about the negative things in their lives, they tend to keep coming up with more negative things to add to that list long after they thought they would stop. The same idea applies to gratitude. Once you think of three things that you're grateful for, you'll tend to come up with a few more. Picture it like a ball rolling down a hill—once your mind gets rolling in a certain direction, positive or negative, it tends to keep rolling in that direction and gains momentum as it rolls. Chi Kung involves moving energy through your entire body. Your mind has an influence on what kind of energy is circulated. If your mind is focused on the negative when you practice Chi Kung, then you will circulate that negativity. And, of course, the reverse is also true.

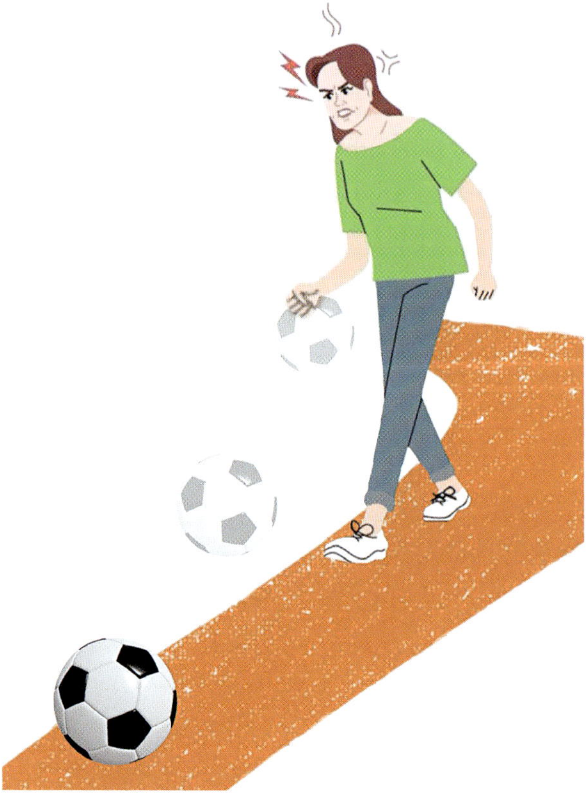

Fig. 5.1. When you practice Chi Kung while your mind is on a negative roll, your body goes along for the ride.

In hypnosis, the word *anchor* is used to capture the experience of establishing a connection between one word, phrase, signal, or action and another, even if they are not the only possible connections that could be made to those things. For example, when people hear the words "Who ya gonna call?" many people still think of the movie *Ghostbusters*. That movie was made decades ago, but the connection is still strong in people's minds. People in recovery can use anchors like this to help them strengthen their commitment to recovery. After performing each of the practices in this book, say to yourself something to the effect of *Each time I do this practice, my recovery and my commit-*

ment to it becomes stronger and stronger; or *Each time I do this practice, the idea of feeding my addiction makes me sick to my stomach*; or *Each time I do this practice, I am reminded of how good it feels to be in recovery.*

SELF-CONTROL AND RELAXATION

Someone dealing with addiction has gotten used to operating with high levels of stress due to the chaos and drama that go with addiction. When they enter recovery, their body is still vigilant, always on guard for more trouble. They may not even be aware of it because they are used to that level of stress. Even if the person is aware of it, they will often complain that despite their best efforts they still cannot relax. They try to meditate, but their mind wanders, and sometimes unwanted thoughts and feelings flood their mind as soon as their guard is down.

This is what makes Chi Kung practices different. The practices keep your mind active while at the same time you relax. Put on some loose clothing, something not too tight around the waist, and we will get started with a few very simple practices.

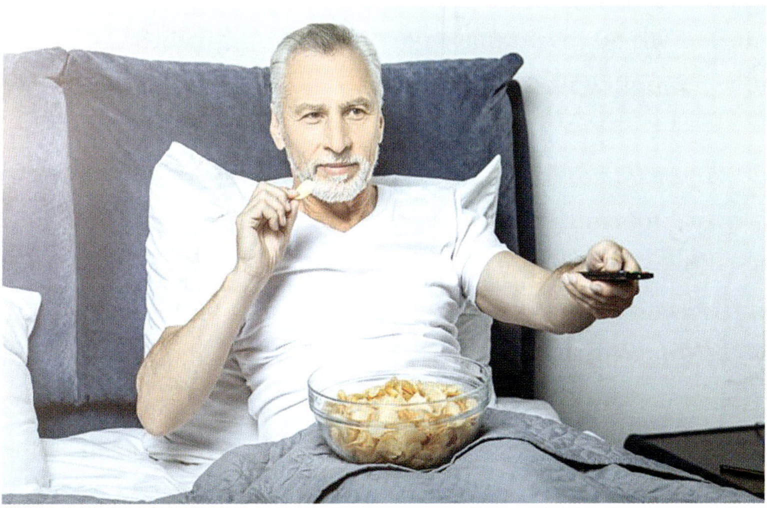

Fig. 5.2. Take time to absorb the benefits between practices. Rest, but do not "retox" your system.

Preparatory Practice

For the seated Chi Kung practices you should be sitting on the edge of a stable chair. When you sit on the edge you are able to receive more energy from the ground below you. Sitting completely still for extended periods of time has become a problem for many people today now that we rely so much on smartphones, tablets, and computers to accomplish so many of our tasks. Do not be a "sitting duck." It is not a good idea to sit still for extended periods of time during the day, as your energy will stagnate and become polluted just like a pool in a forest where the water has stopped flowing. Resting and recharging are important. Sitting and "vegging out" for too long will create problems.

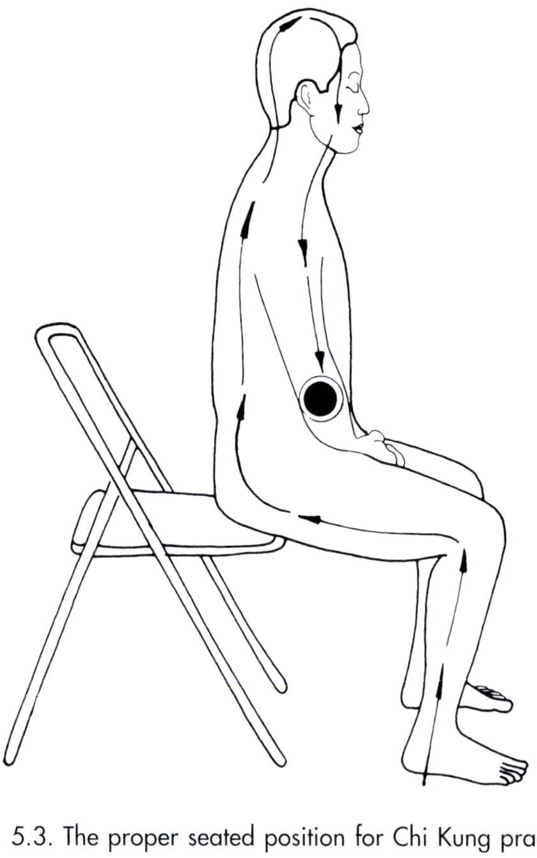

Fig. 5.3. The proper seated position for Chi Kung practice.

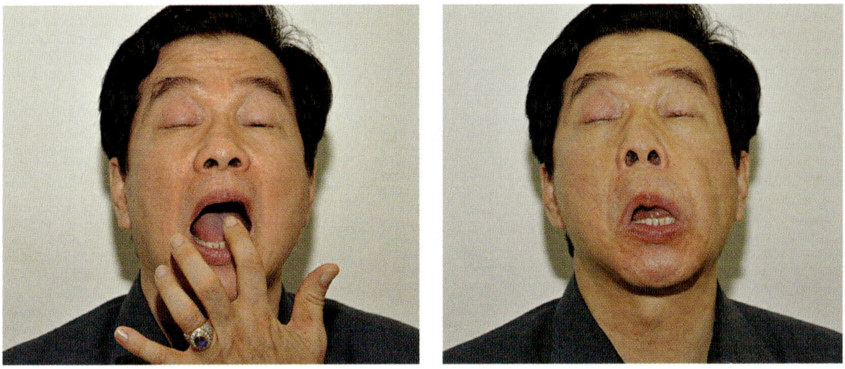

Fig. 5.4. Place your tongue on the roof of your mouth.

1. Place your feet flat on the floor so that you can receive energy from the earth, and so that you do not lose energy out of your feet. Clasp your hands in your lap so that you are not losing energy out of your palms. Lightly touch the tip of your tongue to the roof of your mouth just behind your upper gum line; you will feel a small divot in your palate there, and when your tongue touches that spot it might even taste like you're putting your tongue on the charge points of a battery. Having your tongue there will prevent you from losing energy between the two halves of your jaw. Now you have a complete connected circuit between you and the ground below you.
2. Smile, even if you have to force a smile in the beginning. Lift the corners of your mouth and eyes so that you have a slight grin on your face, like the Mona Lisa. Let the warmth of your smile move through your face and into your body.
3. Now imagine that there is a thread tied to the crown of your head that extends up to the North Star. That thread pulls your spine up and creates a bit more separation between your vertebrae. Tuck your chin in lightly.
4. Slowly rock from side to side on your sitting bones. Think of yourself as being a big glass of water and you are trying to swish the

water enough to wash the insides of the glass with it. You may have the urge to laugh as you do this. Go ahead. Laughing produces good energy. Moving this way might remind you of swaying to music or rocking when you were impatient for class to be over when you were in grade school. It is something we do naturally to feel good. Rock for at least one minute. Then rest and notice how you feel. You will probably feel more alert, lighter, and more relaxed. Rocking on your sitting bones might feel a little uncomfortable at first, as the area around those bones might feel tight. However, rocking this way will eventually loosen those tissues and allow energy to move more freely through your pelvic floor.

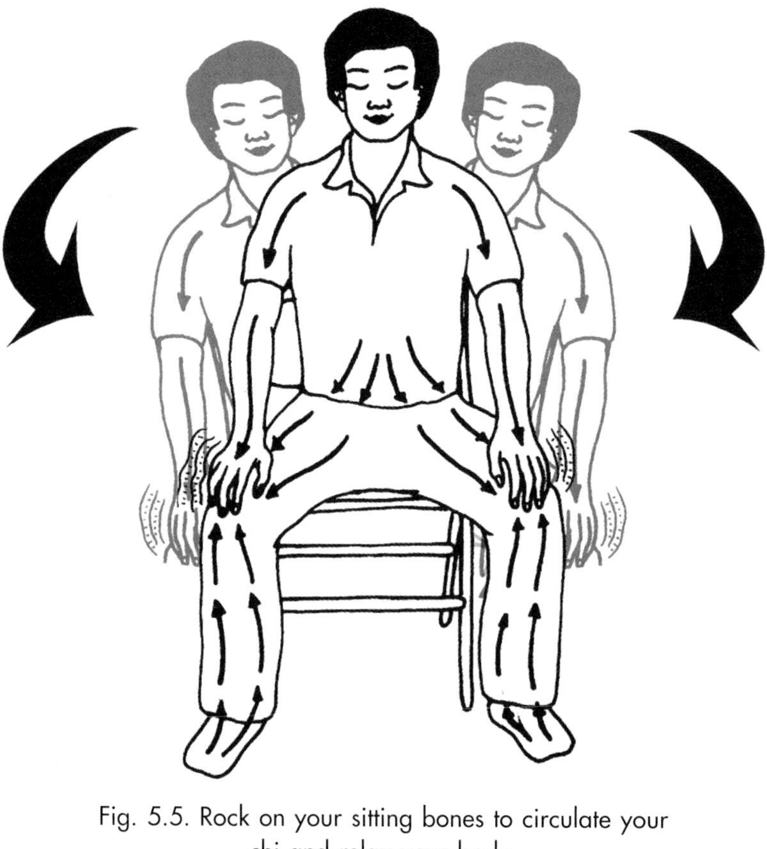

Fig. 5.5. Rock on your sitting bones to circulate your chi and relax your body.

5. Now place your hands, one palm on top of the other, on your lower abdomen. Slowly and lightly move your palms in small circles that get slightly bigger with each rotation, like a spiral. Men should spiral in a clockwise direction, women in a counterclockwise direction. Move slowly enough that you can follow the motions in your mind. Keep spiraling your hands until you have covered your entire lower abdomen. Aim for thirty-six rotations. Then reverse the direction and pack chi in by slowly moving your palms from big circular

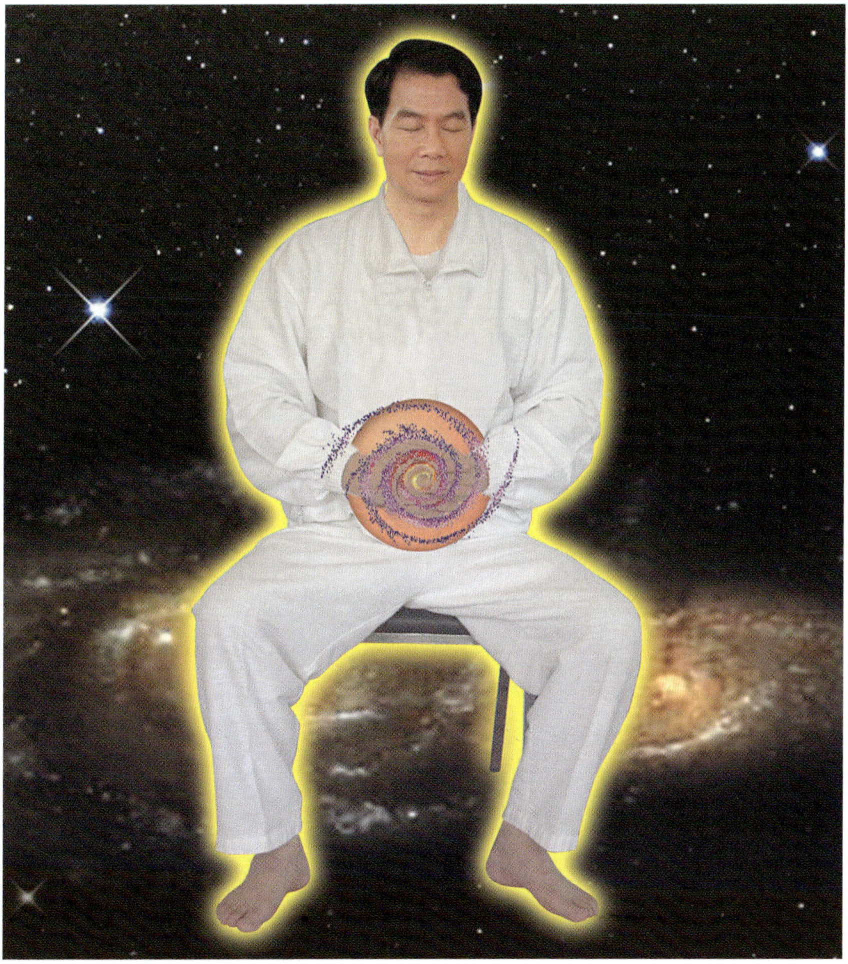

Fig. 5.6. Spiral your chi for relaxation.

motions to progressively smaller ones. Aim for twenty-four rotations. Now rest. Feel the energy moving in your abdomen and flowing out to the rest of your body.

6. Approximately two finger-widths below your navel and three finger-widths inside your abdomen is your Lower Tan Tien, your main major energy source or battery. This is called the Center of Control in the Universal Healing Tao. Focusing your mind on that area, thereby bringing chi to it, allows you to connect with it and adds to its energy. When you are focused on that area you can feel more of a sense of control over your mind, your urges, and your mood. Try it. Put your hands there, one palm on top of the other, and breathe gently but fully into that area. Breathe slowly and gently enough that you do not make any audible sound. Remember to smile. Focus on your Lower Tan Tien and then let your mind drift inside. Think about your organs inside like planets, and your Lower Tan Tien as the sun that they orbit. Explore your inner universe. Notice how quickly you relax and how nice it feels to turn your mind inward. External entertainment may seem appealing, but internal focus can create more reliable and lasting relaxation and enjoyment, and it's free.
7. Once you have achieved the desired state, try to move through your day in sync with that feeling after you get up. Practice carrying that peaceful spirit through your day. Over time you will get better and better at maintaining it and at noticing when you have lost touch with it.

Listen to Your Gut

We've all heard it said, "Listen to your gut." Why do we say that? How come no one suggests that we should listen to our elbows or some other body part? We all seem to know that the gut seems to have access to a source of wisdom that we cannot access any other way. In active addiction people get out of the habit of listening to their gut, which is to say their instincts. Instead, they medicate their bad feelings whenever they feel the need. Even if they try to listen to their gut it probably does not have useful suggestions because it has been so heavily polluted. Once you start recovery it's time to start listening to your gut again.

Smiling to your Lower Tan Tien will allow you to reconnect with your instinctual nature. With practice you can also think while focusing on your gut. You will come up with more effective solutions to your life situations if you do so. We know now that there are neurons in your large intestine, which is why it's called the second brain. The vagus nerves connect the second brain to the brain in your head. If you focus on your Lower Tan Tien, you can do much more than just think about your problems—you can access your feelings and intuition as well, which will provide you with more well-considered solutions. The brain just uses logic and rationality. It is best suited to grocery lists and math problems.

Three Minds into One Mind

Sometimes people have trouble bringing their focus down to their Lower Tan Tien. They are so accustomed to focusing on what's up in their heads that it's difficult to focus anywhere else. Moreover, life during active addiction involves an artificial way of controlling one's feelings by constant thinking, which gets the person out of the habit of paying attention to what is really happening inside of them—how they *feel* as opposed to what they're *thinking*. This practice provides a method to systematically shift the focus from your head to your Lower Tan Tien. Each of the three "minds"—the head, the heart, and the abdomen—contains neurons. Each center experiences a different way of perceiving the world. Combining their energies can provide a way to stay relaxed but maintain one's perspective.

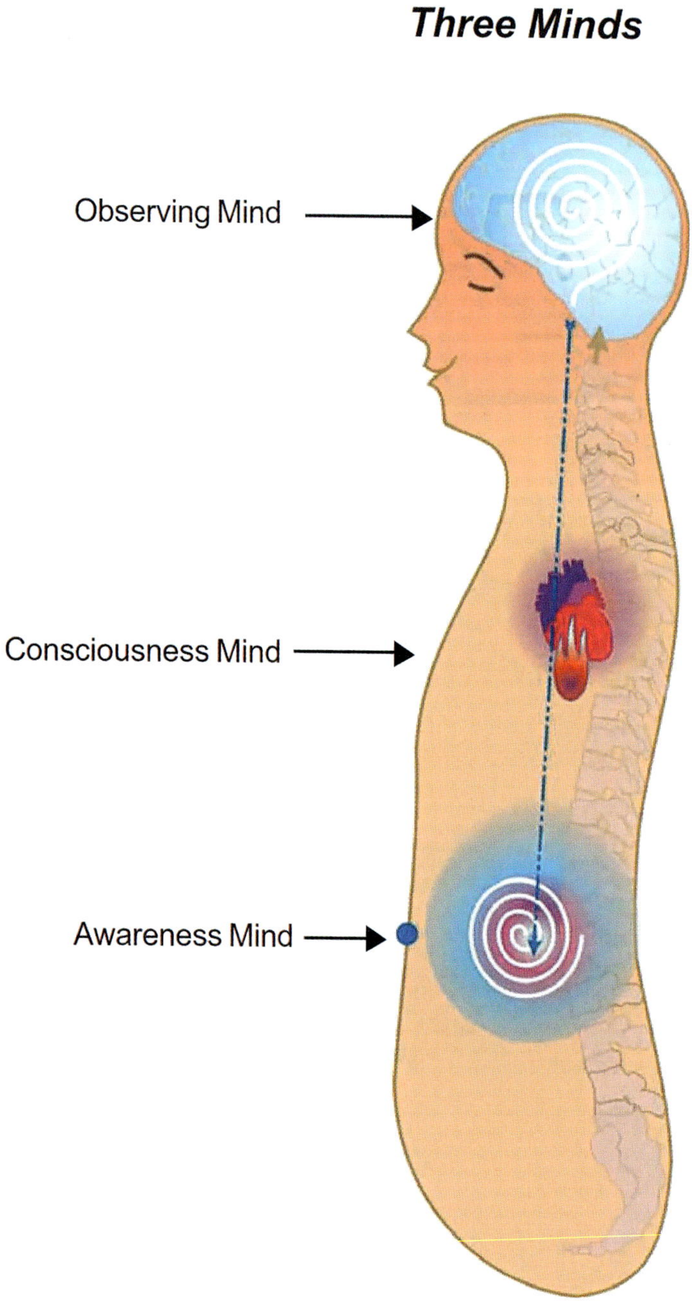

Fig. 5.7. Three Minds into One Mind practice

1. While seated on the edge of a chair as directed above, gently place your fingers on the middle of your forehead. The area behind your fingers is your first mind. In Taoism it is called the Center of Happiness. Smile, breathe, and focus on the area inside your head that is directly behind your fingers. As you focus there, visualize your chi growing and spreading in that area.
2. Now slowly move your fingers down the middle of your face and across your nose, lips, and chin. Move slowly enough that you can follow the movement of your fingers with your mind. Move your fingers down your neck, to the left, and down to your heart, which is your second mind. Bring the energy from the first mind down with your fingers and blend it with the energy around your heart, which is called the Center of Peace. The sac around your heart, the pericardium, contains neurons. Smile, breathe, and focus on your heart. Feel the energy of the two minds growing and spreading through your torso and into your limbs.
3. Smile, breathe, and slowly draw your fingers from your heart back to the center line of your body and then down to your Lower Tan Tien. Bring the energy from the other two minds to your Lower Tan Tien, your third mind, the Center of Control. Blend their energy with the energy there. Focus on that area. Notice that your hands quickly become warm. Feel the energy and warmth grow and spread throughout your body.

Laughing Chi Kung

Laughing Chi Kung can be a powerful way to relax and reset. Many people only laugh when something or someone makes them laugh. However, when life is difficult, it may be quite a long time before we have a chance to laugh. Most of us can remember a time when we had an unexpected big belly laugh with a friend that completely changed the complexion of our day. Everything felt lighter and easier. In recovery, people typically feel shame and may hesitate to laugh until they have cleaned up the mess that their addiction has created. However, that mess is usually pretty big and will take quite a while to clean up. Persevering in recovery will be easier if we laugh through the difficult times. People who go to their first 12-Step meeting are often surprised at the amount of laughter in the meeting. On an intuitive level it seems like people realize that laughter is an essential part of healing. When we're too serious we're told to "lighten up." Dropping the burden of seriousness just feels good, and we all know from personal experience that it is more difficult to focus on negative thoughts when we laugh. We also know from any number of studies that the body's chemistry changes when we laugh. Powerful hormones are released that buffer us from pain and stress. A common saying is "Laughter is the best medicine." Laughing Chi Kung harnesses the power of laughter and uses it to your advantage.

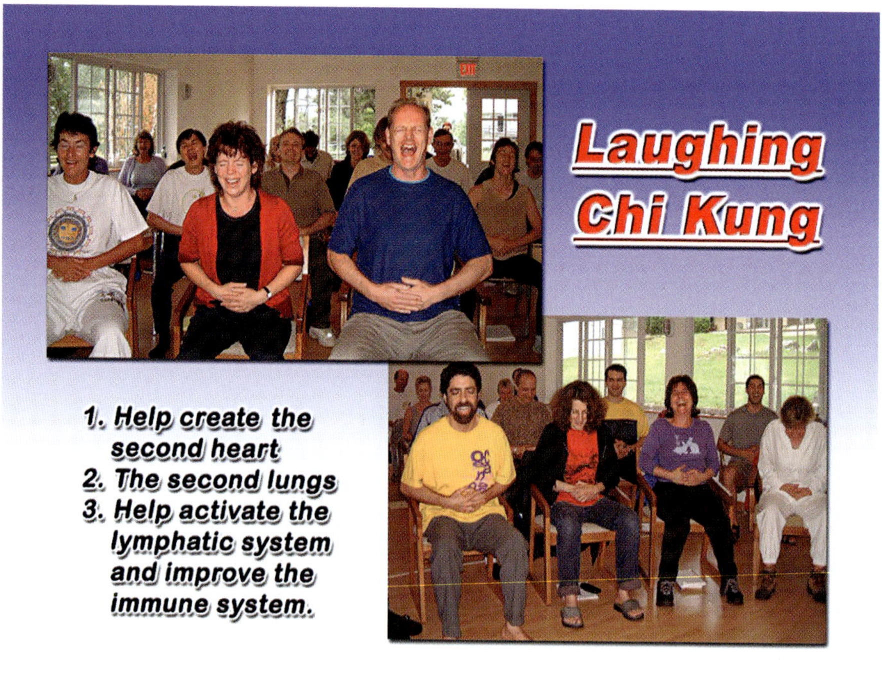
Laughing
Chi Kung
1. Help create the
second heart
2. The second lungs
3. Help activate the
lymphatic system
and improve the
immune system.

Fig. 5.8. Laughing Chi Kung practice.

1. Stand with your feet shoulder-width apart, knees slightly bent. Lightly press the tips of your fingers at the level of your thymus gland, just below your sternum notch.
2. Now laugh loudly and press on that spot with your fingers with each laugh. The initial laugh will likely be forced and artificial, but eventually it becomes more genuine. When you place your fingers on a specific area on your body, you are directing the chi that is produced from laughing to that place. Putting your fingers on your thymus gland helps to activate the killer T-cells, boosting your immune system to push cold and flu bugs out. The effect of shaking the thymus gland is as if you were to shake a hornets' nest to release all the hornets. Placing your fingers in your navel and then giggling can activate the stem cells and push cold and flu bugs out of that area. Placing your fingers on your thigh bones and laughing hard can push toxins out of those bones. As you touch your thigh bones, think about the bones becoming happy and laughing as you laugh out loud.

Self-Love

Many people who seek treatment for their addictions are aware that they do not love themselves. Thinking about all the lying, cheating, or stealing they did while they were actively using leads them to feel shame. The belief that goes along with shame is: "I am bad." How can someone possibly love themselves in recovery, then? Often people will learn how to use daily affirmations to combat their shameful feelings and condemning beliefs. They will repeat over and over things like: "I am a good person." "I deserve to be happy." "I am loveable." Those efforts are not wasted, but their benefit may be limited or temporary if they are not supported by heartfelt feelings. Competing negative self-judgments tend to come quickly to mind and cancel the effects of the affirmations.

Another useful strategy that people usually learn in recovery is to separate their intentions from their addictions. They will remind themselves that they do not act or think the same way when they are not in active addiction. Again, if their hearts are not in this, then those thoughts do not fully translate to the rest of their bodies and especially to their feelings.

As mentioned earlier, in the Universal Healing Tao system the heart is considered to be the Center of Peace. The virtues associated with the heart are love, joy, and happiness. Love comes from the heart, not the mind. Perhaps it is easy to understand, then, why it is important to use the chi from our hearts to enhance our love for ourselves and others. See for yourself:

1. Sit on a chair in the way described earlier. Smile. Turn the corners of your mouth and eyes up in a gentle grin. Human beings are built to be consistent. When we smile, even if it is forced in the beginning, the mind will start searching for positive ideas to support that smile and at the same time it will keep negative thoughts at bay. Just like when we laugh, when we smile, good internal chemical reactions occur that help to relax us and protect us from stress and pain.
2. Now breathe gently but fully into your abdomen and focus on your heart. Visualize a red aura around it. Do not be too concerned if you do not see your heart or the red color clearly, just do what you can. Even if you can see your heart, it may look dark and cloudy at first. The more you smile and focus on it, the clearer and brighter the red aura around your heart will become. Place your hands on your heart if that helps you to focus there. Feel the warmth coming from your heart as you focus on it. As you smile and breathe and focus on your heart, you are transforming the toxic energy in it, emotionally changing impatience, hastiness, hatred, or cruelty into joy, happiness, and love. You will likely start to feel peaceful after a while. Now would be a good time to repeat your affirmations or remind yourself of the difference between your intentions and your addiction. Your internal energy system is more open to those ideas now.

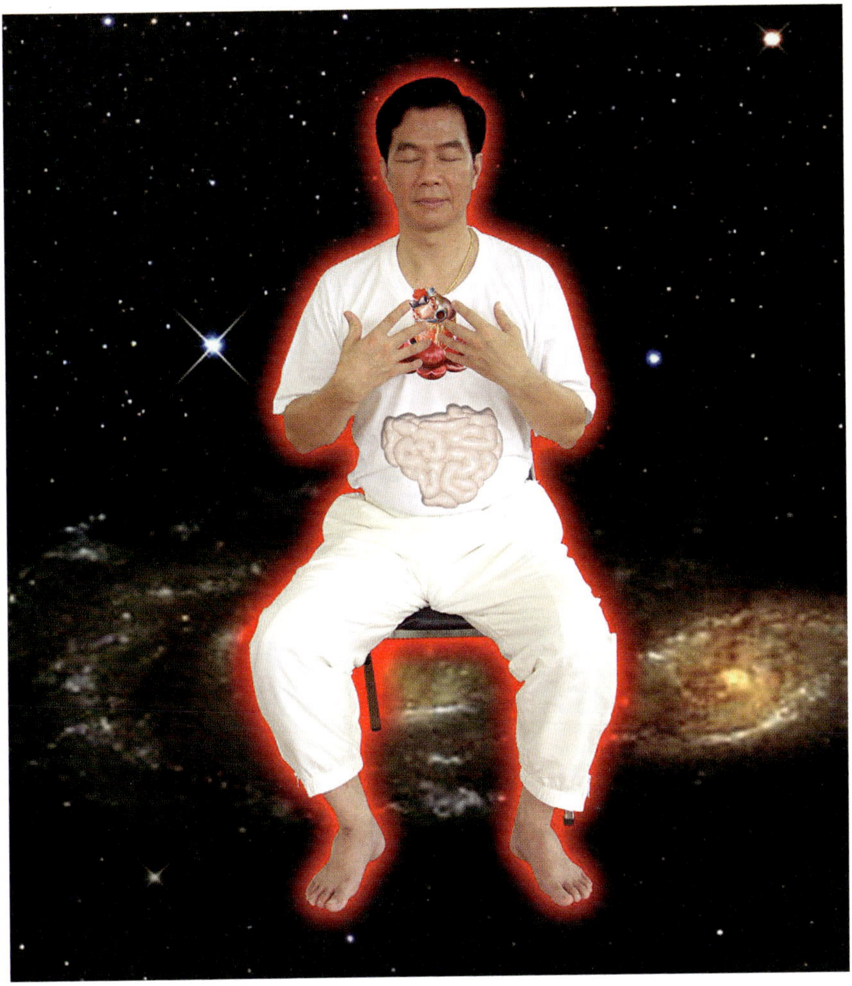

Fig. 5.9. Smile into your heart to increase feelings of self-love.

What you are doing in this simple practice is an act of self-love. Your mind may argue when you try to change your thinking, but your body will not argue when you focus on your heart this way. At first it will probably be necessary to sit and focus on your heart. Eventually, with enough practice, you'll be able to do it even when you're going about your daily activities. Spend one day focusing on this exercise and then see how you feel at the end of the day. That should be enough to convince you to keep practicing.

Increasing Energy

In the Universal Healing Tao system we consider the Lower Tan Tien to be important for a number of reasons. As noted earlier, it is our major energy source. It is also the source of what is considered to be our "gut instinct." Chi can be stored there, and because it is located in the middle of the body it helps us feel more balanced and centered when we focus on it. And one of the greatest benefits of focusing on your Lower Tan Tien is the increased energy it can bring.

1. In a seated position, place your palms one on top of the other and over your Lower Tan Tien.
2. Smile, breathing naturally, and keep focusing on the Lower Tan Tien for thirty-six or even seventy-two breaths. Try to see a ball of energy spinning inside your lower abdomen.

You will probably notice that now you have energy that will last for hours. Notice that you can feel relaxed but also have energy at the same time when you practice like this. That is the balance that people are often seeking in life. In active addiction, people often alternate between uppers and downers in an attempt to create a similar effect. Smiling to your Lower Tan Tien does not create such drastic mood swings; it doesn't lead you to act in ways that you will regret later, and it doesn't cost you anything.

How to Stop Worrying and Ruminating

Sometimes you will hear people saying something like, "If only I could turn my brain off once in a while, it just goes and goes." They try meditation apps and breathing exercises and still cannot stop their minds from whizzing around various topics. Notice that your brain stops thinking about so many things while you are focusing on your Lower Tan Tien. There are several explanations for why that happens. One reason is because you are busy and engaged. Focusing on your Lower Tan Tien and smiling and breathing takes concentration. By doing this, you do not have enough attention left over for other, less helpful thoughts. Another reason why it creates a quiet mind is because by bringing your focus down your body to your Lower Tan Tien, you are taking your focus off of your head. There's an old Taoist saying, "Where the mind goes, the chi follows." By doing this, your brain gets a chance to cool off and recharge.

Yet another reason why focusing this way is helpful is because it does not trigger unwanted thoughts. With good intentions, people often tell themselves to stop worrying. The trouble with that approach is that the deeper part of the mind, where automatic thoughts and urges begin, uses pictures as its language. When people tell themselves to stop worrying, that deeper part of their mind needs a picture to understand what has been suggested. It will need to know what they want to stop worrying about so it can understand the command. That requires picturing the worry first and then trying to stop thinking about it. This all happens in an instant. People end up unintentionally triggering their worries. If you want proof of this, try telling yourself not to think about a banana. See what happens? Besides, just thinking something like "Stop worrying" is giving another thought to add to the jumble in an already busy mind.

6

Practices for Detoxification and Unwinding the Body

When someone is in active addiction there's a lot of stress that comes with the territory as a result of having to hide their problem, lie about it, keep track of all the lies, and try to stay one step ahead of the mounting consequences of all of this. There can be consequences with family and romantic relationships, financial consequences, and health consequences. Even after the person stops feeding their addiction, there are still consequences that must be addressed. They often have to deal with debts, resentments and judgments from friends and family, and a large to-do list of tasks that did not get taken care of that accumulated while they were too focused on medicating their feelings.

When we feel stressed, we often end up with tightness in the upper back and neck, and this impedes the flow of the energy that travels up the spine to the brain. The following three Chi Kung practices restore the flow of chi to the brain.

Crane Neck

When we do not get enough energy traveling up to the brain as a result of the physical tension caused by stress, it's hard to think quickly, clearly, and effectively. "Brain fog" is a common complaint. People sometimes try to stretch their neck out by bending it to each side; however, stretching that way does not do much to loosen up the lower back. And it may stretch too much to one side, which can lead to more tension and pain. The Crane Neck is a Chi Kung practice that can gently and safely relieve the tension in your neck and upper back and thereby restore your ability to think clearly.

1. Sit on the edge of a sturdy chair with your feet on the floor. Place your hands on top of your legs near your knees. Jut your chin out. Then reach forward gently with your chin and allow your body to follow. Your body will move in a curved trajectory, moving forward and then down.
2. When your lower back has moved forward as much as comfortably possible, gently tuck your chin in so that it presses back toward your neck. Keep it there as you straighten back up to an upright seated position. This movement allows your neck to stretch out as the movement of your chin opens up the neck region at the sides and down to your upper back as it presses against your neck. Practice the Crane Neck a few times a day to keep your neck and upper back loose. Then energy can travel easily up your spine to your brain.
3. Rest.

Practicing Crane Neck a few times a day will slowly correct the curvature of your neck that causes tightness and will restore a good flow of chi to your brain.

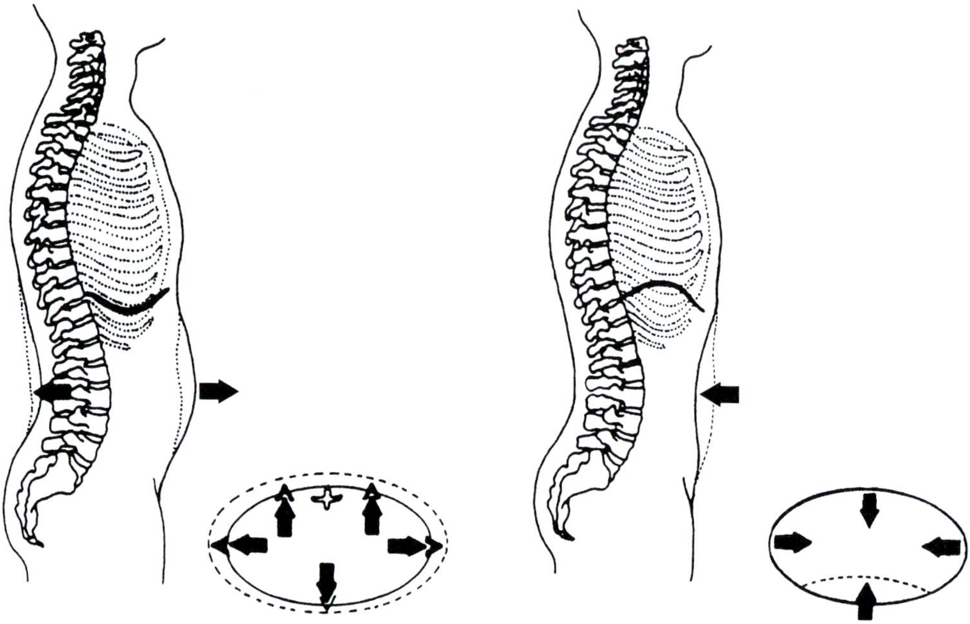

Fig. 6.1. Practice the Crane Neck a few times a day to keep your neck and upper back loose. Then energy can travel easily up your spine to your brain.

Spinal Cord Breathing

Spinal Cord Breathing is a practice that flexes the joints in the spine, allowing spinal cord fluid to flow between the vertebrae to lubricate them, opening the sacral and cranial pumps and flushing the cerebrospinal fluid and chi up the spine. The brain is energized as a result.

1. Stand with your feet shoulder-width apart and your knees slightly bent. Bend your arms at the elbows and make loose fists with your hands.
2. Raise your arms so that your fists are at the height of your nose and the palm sides of your fists are pointed toward you. Your elbows should be at a lower height than your hands. Relax your shoulders.
3. Now keep your elbows down and pull your fists out to each side of your body. As your fists move to the sides, tilt your head back

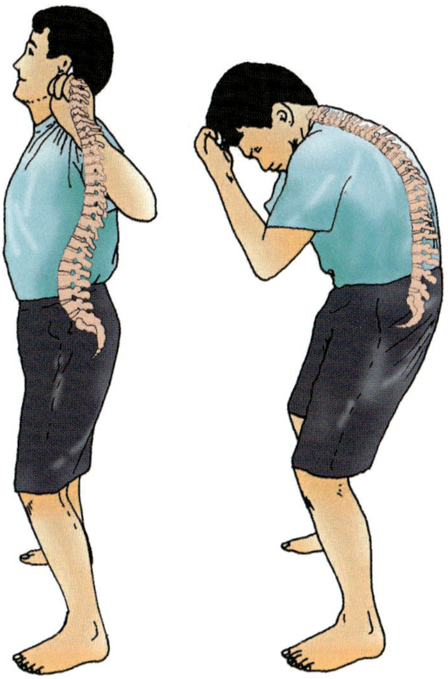

Fig. 6.2. Spinal Cord Breathing flushes energy up the spine and into the brain.

and flex your lower back so that your buttocks lift up. Your spine should look like it is in a backward *C* shape from a side view. Do not tighten. Just flex the spine. If you tighten too much the fluid and energy cannot flow properly.

4. Now reverse the *C* shape in your spine. Gently roll your head forward and down to tuck your chin into your neck. Flex your lower back in the other direction so that your tailbone moves forward and tucks in.
5. Slowly move back and forth between these two positions nine times. Proper breathing for this practice will happen naturally. You will breathe in as you pull your elbows back and breathe out when you curl your body forward. Think about your body filling up with a shimmering golden energy when you breathe in, and dark, gray, cloudy energy coming out of the pores of your entire body as you breathe out.
6. Rest.

Shaking to Let Go

When your friends and loved ones are trying to support you after something upsetting has happened, they will often encourage you to "just let it go." They probably do not want you to feel bad for any longer than necessary. The intention is to be supportive, but sometimes letting go is not so easy. Some things that happen are too weird or too awful and cannot be easily understood or fixed. Then your mind tends to search for a different perspective or a solution that will allow you to stop thinking about it, but to no avail. Without another option for addressing the issue you can end up feeling stuck in kind of a loop in which your mind is fixated on finding a way out of the situation. A common expression in these kinds of situations is the advice to "just shake it off." Why do we say that? On some level we must recognize that the upset energy is stuck inside, and that moving it enough might dislodge it and allow it to release, freeing up the mind so that clear thinking is restored. Taoist Chi Kung practitioners have been using shaking for millennia. Not only does it help us let go of stuck and upset feelings, it also moves energy rapidly throughout the whole body if it is done correctly, and as a bonus it pushes toxins out through the skin. Try it.

1. Stand with your feet shoulder-width apart. Bend your knees slightly but not too much. You should still be able to see your toes when you look down. Move your arms far enough away from your body that there are spaces the size of a ping-pong ball between the inside of your arms and your armpits.
2. Now shake and bounce your whole body. Move every part of your body, especially the parts that tend to feel tight like your jaws, hips, and ankles. You might want to open your mouth and make a sound like *aaaaaaaaaa* as you do this. Keep bouncing and shaking for at least one minute. Then slowly come to a stop.
3. Notice what you feel in your hands. That tingling is your chi. Notice how light you feel. Practicing shaking and bouncing can help you to

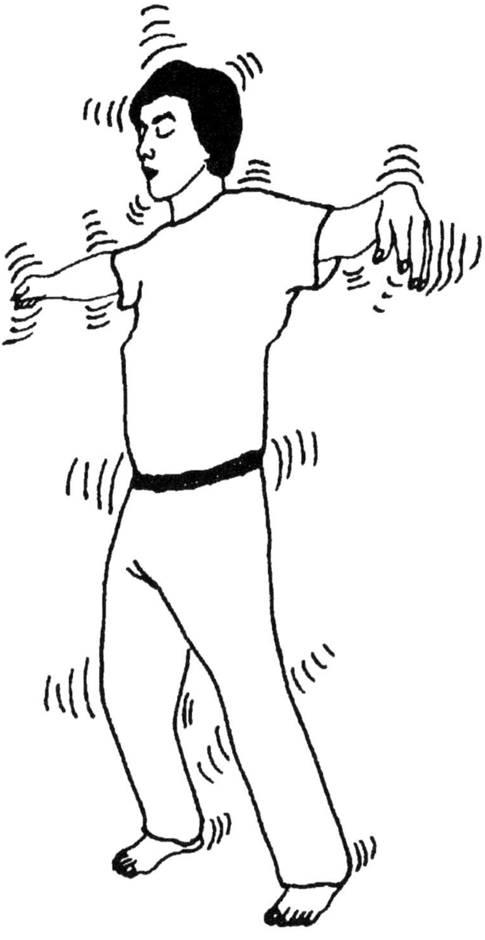

Fig. 6.3. Shaking your body helps you take your focus off of whatever issue is bothering you.

shift out of a negative mindset and move on to a more positive and productive day. Only perform this practice during the day, as it is too stimulating to do close to bedtime.

STRETCHING YOUR STRESS OUT

People in recovery are no strangers to chronic stress. Their compromised state while in active addiction created lots of problems, and they usually have a big pile of them to sort out once they enter recovery. As a result, they often struggle with how to unwind without resorting to whatever they were addicted to. They may try various kinds of meditations, but these will have limited success. The reason is not that meditation is not helpful—it's because meditation practices rarely treat the psoas muscles. Most people have a tight psoas and rarely know it. Tao Yin is a set of practices in the Universal Healing Tao System that focus on restoring the body back to health. Within Tao Yin there are several movements that specifically teach people how to stretch and strengthen their psoas muscles. The following exercise, Monkey Clasps Knees, is one of them.

Monkey Clasps Knees

The psoas muscles lie on either side of the lower spine (lumbar area) and run through your pelvis to the top of your femur (thigh bone). You use them to move your lower back, hips, and legs. These are the muscles that tighten when you feel stressed. The leg muscles and tendons will

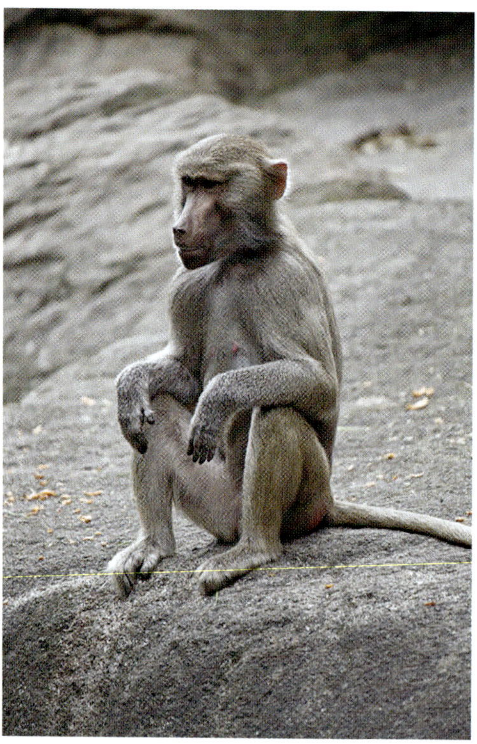

Fig. 6.4. A monkey instinctively stretches its psoas.

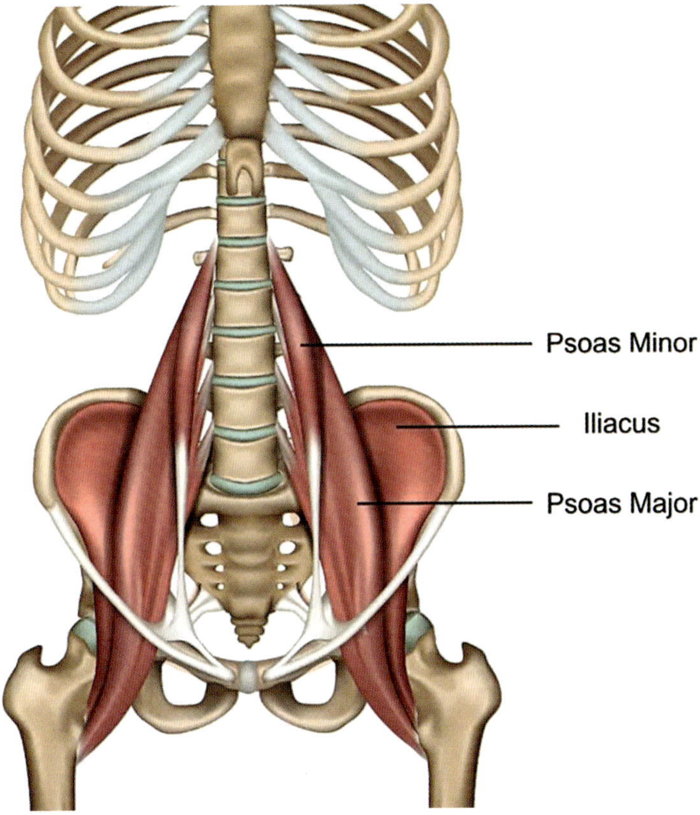

Fig. 6.5. The psoas muscles.

only stretch to a limited extent as long as the psoas muscles are still tight. They will stay tight for as long as it takes for you to effectively stretch and strengthen them. Until then, you will tend to feel on edge. Having a "happy" psoas means you'll feel more grounded and relaxed, and physically you'll have a bigger range of movement.

1. Lie flat on your back on a mat. Breathe naturally. Imagine that as you inhale you are drawing golden, shimmering energy into your whole body. When you exhale, visualize dark, gray, or cloudy toxins coming out of your body through your skin and going into the ground around you to be recycled. Breathe like that until you feel relaxed and comfortable.

2. Slowly bend your legs at the knees and raise your feet off the mat so that your shins are parallel with the mat. Raise your head off the mat just enough so that your chin can lightly tuck into your neck. Now your spine is elongated. Your back should be flat against the mat and your neck in line with your spine.
3. Wrap your arms around your knees and clasp your fingers together so that your two hands are joined together around your knees. Now slowly press your knees up as if you are trying to press them against your entwined hands. This creates a counterpressure between your hands and knees. That pressure forces your psoas muscles to stretch to adjust your body to the movement. Breathe while you hold this posture, and hold it for six breaths.

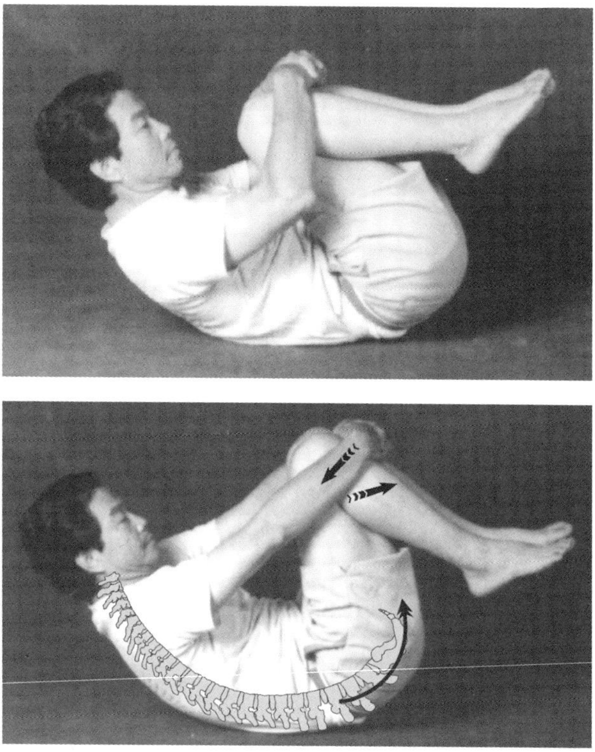

Fig. 6.6. The Monkey Clasps Knees exercise torques and strengthens the psoas muscles.

4. Unclasp your hands, lower your legs and head, and relax. Breathe in golden energy, breathe out dark and cloudy toxins. Keep doing that until your body has completely relaxed.
5. Repeat this sequence two more times.

DEEP CLEANSING

The longer toxins stay in your system, the deeper they will embed. Eventually they will get into your bones and organs. Stopping an addiction is not the entire detoxification process, as the effects of the toxins will still be in the body. This is true not just for those suffering from an addition—we all accumulate toxins. They come to us through the air we breathe, the things we eat and drink, and the emotional effects that others have on us. Taoist Chi Kung is an ancient personal recycling program. We need to regularly recycle our internal garbage. The following two practices facilitate the removal of toxins, both physical and emotional.

Detoxification Chi Kung

A practice from the Iron Shirt Chi Kung tradition involves hitting and slapping the body all over, which not only helps to release toxins but also stimulates the stem cells. This practice is traditionally done with a bamboo hitter that has twenty-five strands fastened to the handle,* but the practice is just as effective if you use your hands. You spread your fingers and keep them somewhat loose so that you can get the same shock-wave effect when your fingers bump against one another when you strike your body as when the bamboo strands bump against one another when you use the hitter. It is very important that the slapping action is gentle enough so as not to cause any bruising or pain, but energetic enough to create vibrations. Note that this practice should be done only during the day as it is very stimulating, and doing it at night might prevent you from falling asleep.

*These can be purchased at the online shop and products page at MantakChia.com.

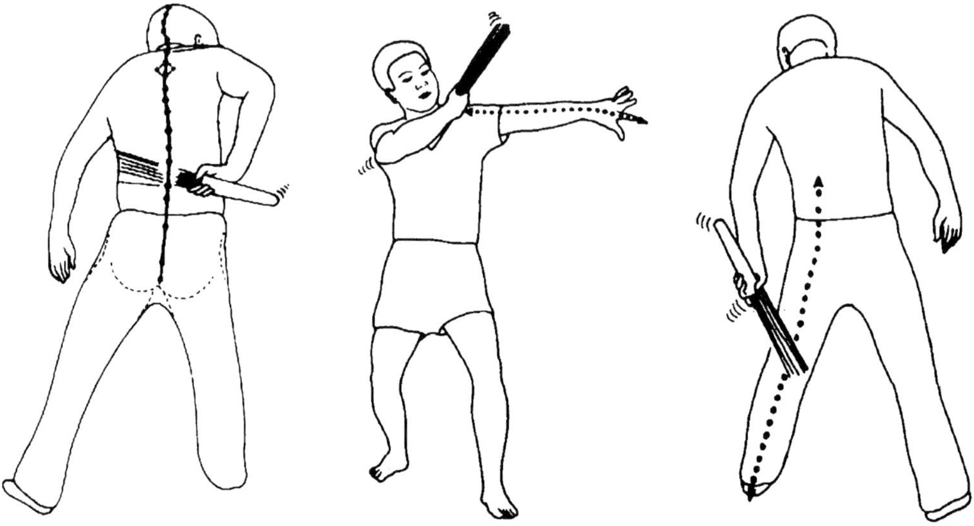

Fig. 6.7. Gently hit your body with a bamboo hitter or with loose fingers to release toxins from your bones and organs.

1. Stand with your feet shoulder-width apart, shoulders relaxed, knees slightly bent and positioned approximately over your toes. The tailbone is slightly tucked, the spine upright.
2. Relax, take a deep breath, and as you exhale, smile.
3. Slowly and gently slap your entire body. If you are going to use your hands to lightly hit your body, rub your palms together to make them warm and energized. Breathe and smile. Gently slap your body all over with your hands while your fingers stay loosely separated, or use a bamboo hitter to do the same. Do not hit yourself too hard. You do not want to do damage. You just want to allow the increasing vibration that is created by doing this to push toxins out through your largest organ, your skin. Slap lightly all over.
4. Stand still and feel your feet connected to the earth and your crown connected to the universe. Take a deep breath and relax. Smile into your heart and feel your heart smiling at you.

Practicing hitting yourself this way will increase the red blood cell count in your bones and increase your bone density. People in recovery often have a desire to beat themselves up emotionally to teach themselves a lesson and change their behavior. The only thing that kind of self-shaming accomplishes is more bad feelings, which creates more toxicity. If you want to beat yourself up, do it gently with a bamboo hitter or your own fingers and stop the cycle of shame.

Opening the Wind Gates

Sick energy is described as wind energy in Taoism. Around the rim of our navels are what are known as the wind gates. They let the wind out of our organs. As we go through life, those gates can close due to stress and physical tension in that area, which creates a buildup of toxins. We need to reopen the wind gates regularly so that they can keep releasing the wind energy from our organs. A practice in the Universal Healing Tao System called Chi Nei Tsang teaches how to open the wind gates.

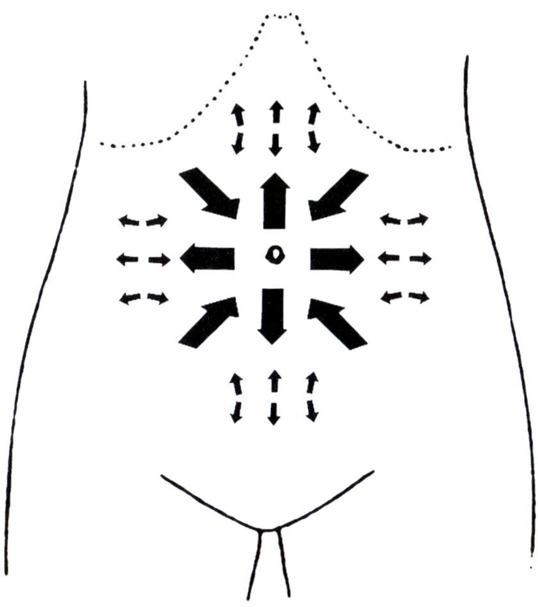

Fig. 6.8. Opening the wind gates lets sick energy out of your body.

1. Before you eat, lie on your back with your legs outstretched. It is easier and more effective to open the wind gates when you do not have a stomach full of food.
2. Use the thumb on one hand to press straight down on the rim of your navel, about half an inch from the center of your navel. Press comfortably as much as you can without feeling pain. Hold your thumb there for about ten seconds. As you press you may feel a pulsing that feels like a heartbeat. If it hurts a bit when you press on that point it will likely hurt less if you do this practice regularly. As your thumb presses down, you are opening that gate and flushing energy to the nearest organ that is in line with that spot. The gate on the left side of your navel points to the left kidney, for example.
3. Once you have finished holding that point for about ten seconds, move your thumb to another point around the rim of your navel and press down on it for another ten seconds. There are eight gates around your navel. They are positioned above, below, to the left, to the right, and at the four diagonal corners. Repeat this process for each of the eight wind gates.
4. Rest. Think of the benefits of this practice as something akin to tuning your car's engine.

LETTING GO OF CONTROL

In active addiction, people become more and more focused on controlling their surroundings so that they can keep feeding their addiction. They need to manipulate and lie and deceive to get people to cover the mistakes they make. They need to convince the people around them that they are fine and do not need to stop using whatever it is they're addicted to. In recovery, the urge to try to control their circumstances does not just go away even after they stop using. This habit may last for quite some time after starting recovery. This can be baffling and upsetting to the loved ones of the person with an addiction—they somehow think that if the addictive behavior stops, then the lying and manipulations will stop, too.

The addict's loved ones—usually family members or very close friends—also tend to have control issues for different reasons. They will worry and try to control things that are beyond their control, which is to say the addictive behavior of their loved one. Their fear for the addicted person and their desire to help them eventually becomes a habit that carries over to other things and people in their lives. This tendency is the hallmark of codependency. At this point the controlling behavior of the person with an addiction and the control pattern of their loved ones starts to collide. Trying to control others and situations is very stressful! Both sides need to remember how freeing it can be to let go of control and embrace life on its own terms. Having a simple way to feel that again is wonderful.

Opening the Door of Life

When we are too rigid and try too hard to control our surroundings, we become physically tense. When we are chronically tense the spine becomes tight. It works the other way, too. If the spine is tight, then we have difficulty responding to life in flexible and adaptable ways. Loosening the spine can help you out of that bind. The practice called Opening the Door of Life helps to loosen the spine so we can let go of controlling behavior.

1. Stand with your feet shoulder-width apart and bend your knees slightly. Keep your shoulders relaxed with a space the size of a ping-pong ball between the inside of your upper arms and your armpits. Your hands are relaxed and down at first.
2. Gently twist your spine and allow one palm to swing forward with the twist and place it gently on your Lower Tan Tien. Put the back of your other hand on your Ming Men, the Door of Life, which is directly opposite your Lower Tan Tien on your back.

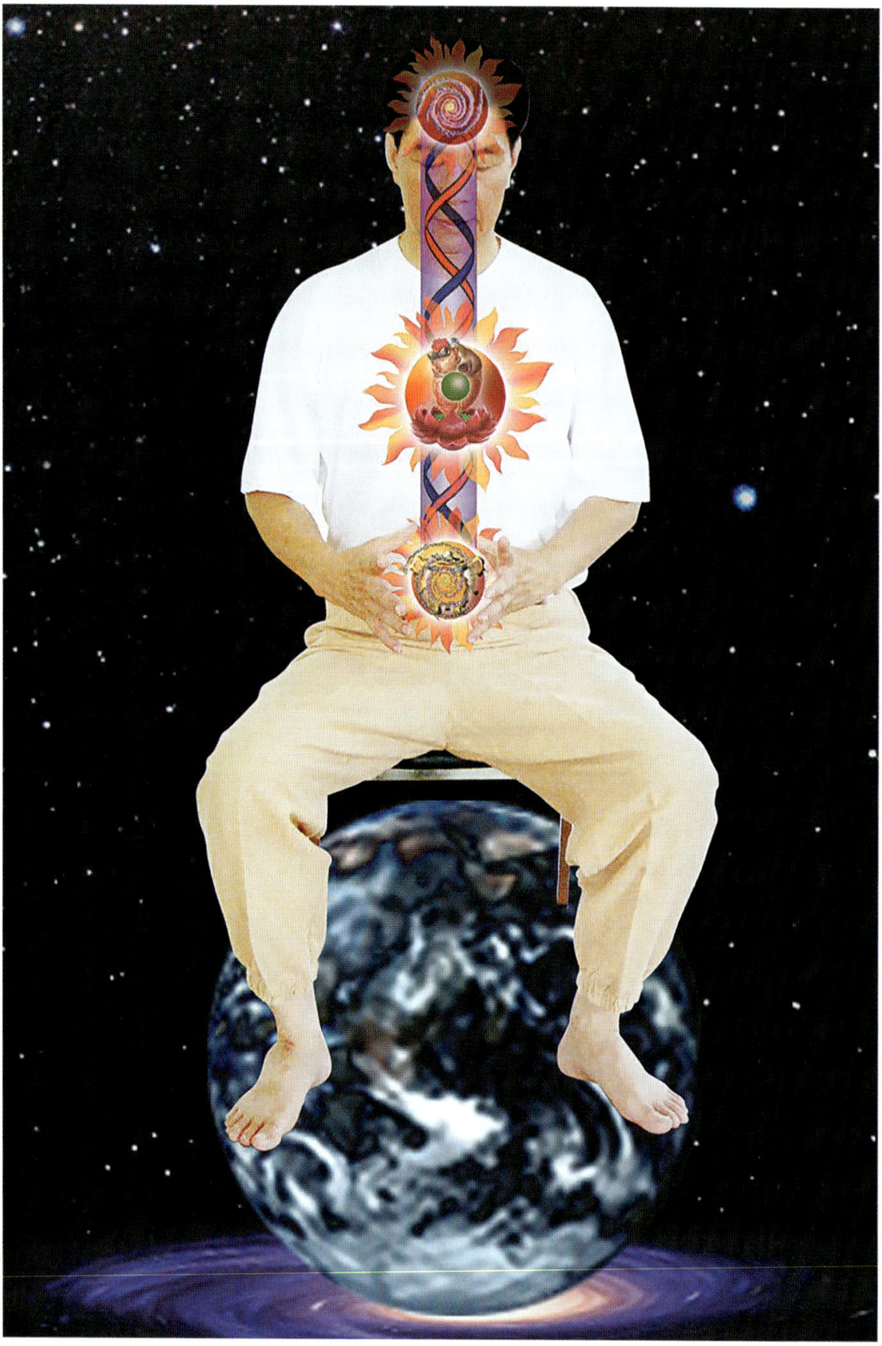

Fig. 6.9. Opening the Door of Life creates more flexibility in your approach to life.

3. Gently twist your spine in the other direction. Do not twist too hard, otherwise you will create more tightness, which will defeat the purpose of this exercise. As you twist, allow your hands to swap positions so that the one that was in front is now on the back and vice versa.
4. As you practice twisting back and forth, the twisting should start mostly from your hands, and the arms will follow the twisting motion. Twist back and forth for at least one minute. You may hear or feel some snapping and popping in your tendons as you practice. This is common. You may notice that this practice accomplishes for your spine what wringing out a wet rag accomplishes for the rag: you are wringing the toxins out of your spine like you would wring water out of a rag; you are also loosening the vertebrae in the spine and allowing more cerebrospinal fluid to flow between them.
5. Rest.

CIRCULATING POSITIVE INTENTIONS THROUGHOUT THE BODY

Masaru Emoto was a Japanese researcher who examined the effects of our words on water. He photographed molecules of frozen water after he said positive or negative things to the water. The water molecules dramatically changed when he did that. His research is found in his best-selling 2005 book *The Hidden Messages in Water*, and it offers insight into the impact of our intentions and thoughtforms, whether positive or negative.

We are two-thirds water. The average human male has about 36 trillion cells. The average female body has about 28 trillion cells. Dr. Emoto's research highlighted the impact that our judgments of ourselves have on our cells. People who have addictions usually carry shame. They have negative beliefs about themselves as a result. The loved ones of the addict tend to believe they should have done more to help or should have realized that help was needed earlier, so they too carry negative beliefs about themselves, usually in the form of guilt. Think about how much these kinds of negative thoughtforms are affecting one's cells. When people have negative beliefs about themselves, they tend to not try as hard because they do not believe they can succeed. Finding a way to change their views of themselves can help them to find the enthusiasm to do their best and get better results.

Charging Your Water Element

This Charging Water exercise helps focus and draw positive energy to you and your cells. Try it.

1. Put an ounce or two of water in a small glass. Hold the glass from the bottom with one hand. Reach up to the heavens with the other

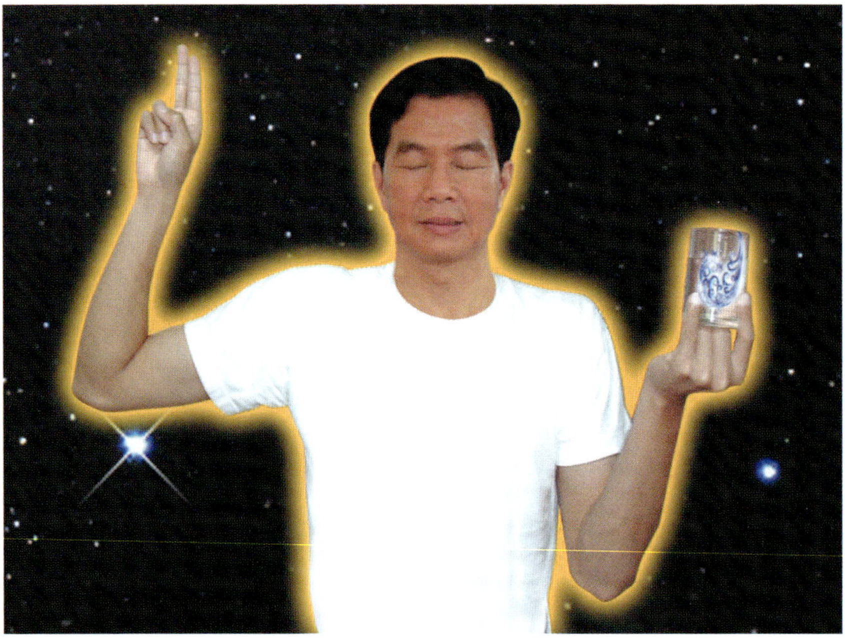

Fig. 6.10. We are two-thirds water, so charging our cells affects how we think about ourselves.

hand while using the sword finger gesture: point your index and middle fingers upright while holding the other three fingers into your palm. Think about connecting the energy from your outstretched fingers up to the North Star and the Big Dipper. Draw that energy down from the stars into your fingers.

2. Repeat these words: "Power comes from the cosmos. Yin has the power to dissolve all the sickness, all the bad energy, and all the bad fortune."
3. Bring your sword fingers down and point them at the rim of the glass. While circling near the rim with your fingers, say, "By my command, please carry out the order now." Then make an *X* over the glass with your fingers. Do it again. Circle the rim of the glass and make an *X* while you repeat the words.

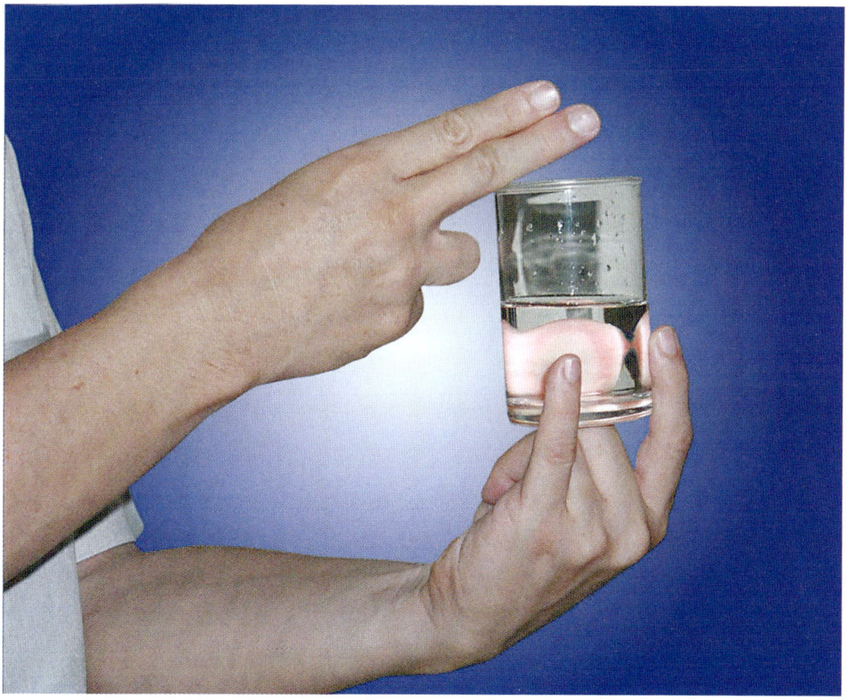

Fig. 6. 11. Charging water with good intentions can change your view of yourself.

4. Reach into the glass near the water level with your sword fingers and think about pulling toxins out of the water as you pull your hand up and out of the glass. Do this a few times. After you pull your hand up out of the glass each time, reach to the side and flick the toxins out of your hands and into the ground to be recycled.
5. Now hold the glass in front of your heart with both hands and say, "This sacred water will give me health, wealth, and longevity." Feel your heart energy charging the water. Now drink the water slowly. Now the good intentions that you projected into the water can be circulated through the cells and tissues of your body.

7

Practices for Self-Confidence

People in recovery often struggle with low self-esteem. Feeling shame about their actions when they were in active addiction usually comes with the belief that they are somehow "bad." They tend to feel like they do not fit in mainstream society. Positive affirmations can be helpful to combat such negative views, but they only last for so long, as the negative feelings and beliefs can return soon after the affirmations are no longer being used. On the other hand, creating a strong, powerful flow of energy in the body is an experience that negative memories and self-limiting beliefs cannot argue with or erase.

STRENGTHENING SELF-DISCIPLINE

A person who tries to refrain from their addiction will often rely on sheer willpower. Actually, a great deal of recovery involves accepting the idea that an addiction can override a person's willpower, even if they're using the strategy of staying away from the people, places, and things that could activate the thoughts and urges that could lead them off-track. The goal of recovery is not to be able to stare into the face of one's addiction and not give in to temptation. Do not try to test the strength of your recovery by challenging yourself to be around triggers and not give in to them. Eventually you will give in to them. That does not prove that you are weak; it just proves that you have an addiction. Nevertheless, willpower is still an important part of what people need in order to stick to their strategies.

Increasing Kidney Chi

The kidneys are the source of willpower. If they are strong, clean, and healthy, and their energy is balanced, then we will have strong willpower. The kidneys are also the organs in which fear, stress, and anxiety are created. As a result, people in recovery often struggle with their willpower because dealing with all the challenges and changes that are required to stay on track is very stressful, which challenges the kidneys. Ironically, the more they put pressure on themselves to stay on track and make all the changes that are required, the more likely their willpower is going to weaken.

Aside from drinking water, there are other things that people can do to make sure their kidney energy is as strong as possible. Rubbing softly on the kidneys can help. As well, gently knocking on the kidneys is another way to make them function better. (See figures 7.1–7.3.) It is important to avoid knocking too hard on them. Kidneys are small, sensitive organs. When we knock on them, we are not trying to hurt them, just wake them up and gently push toxins out. Think about knocking on a screen door to get the dust out of the screen—that's about as hard as you should knock on your kidneys. Many people in recovery have ankle pain, pain in the back of their legs, lower back pain, ringing in their ears, or headaches and receive no help when they see a Western doctor or specialist. That is often because their discomfort is coming from an imbalance in their kidneys.

1. Stand with your feet shoulder-width apart. Bend your knees slightly. Stand on your tiptoes if you can. The kidney meridian extends from the point in the middle of the ball of the foot that touches the ground when you stand on your tiptoes. In acupuncture, this point, Kidney 1, is called the Bubbling Springs point. It extends up along the middle of the balls of the feet to your ankles. It then extends up the back of your legs to your kidneys, and then up your back and neck to the wells underneath the base of your ears.
2. Make loose, soft fists with your hands. Reach behind you with your fists so that your hands are close together in the back. Your knuckles on your index fingers should lightly touch. Now your hands are resting on your kidneys.
3. Rub up and down slowly and gently on your kidney area for about thirty seconds. Rest. When you rub the kidneys they will warm up; blood flow increases, toxins are released, and your willpower increases as a result. You will also feel more lively, as the kidneys are our source of energy.
4. Now you can try gently knocking on your kidneys. Still standing with your feet shoulder-width apart, bend your knees slightly and make loose fists with your hands.
5. Reach behind your back so your fists are resting lightly on your kidneys. Stand on your tiptoes if you can. Take a deep breath into your belly and hold it. That will help you put some padding around your kidneys so that when you knock on them they will have some protection, in a similar way to how airbags protect the passengers in a car.
6. Knock lightly for as long as you can comfortably do so, continuing to hold your breath. Once you start to struggle to hold your breath you can stop knocking on your kidneys, stop standing on your tiptoes, and take a deep breath.
7. Rest.

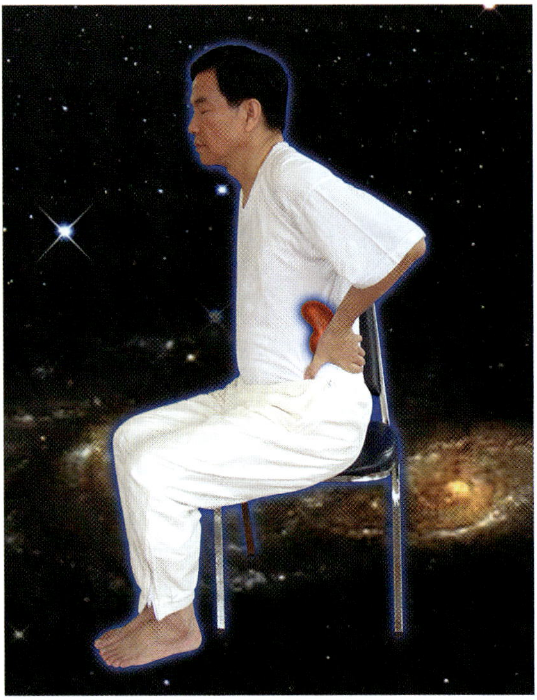

Fig. 7.1. Rubbing on your kidneys activates natural, calm energy.

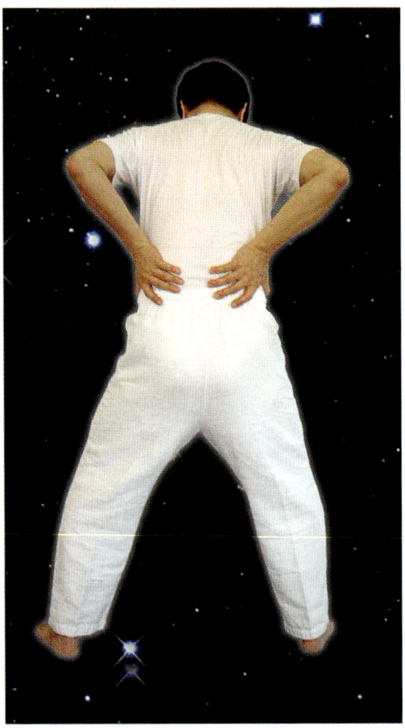

Fig. 7.2. Gently rubbing your kidneys helps to push toxins out and restores your energy.

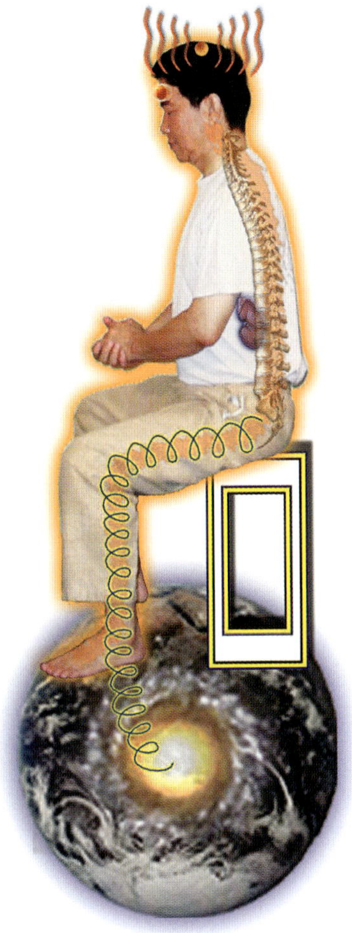

Fig. 7.3. The Bubbling Springs point and the kidney meridian.

Drinking Coffee to Energize?

Think about what happens when people drink coffee to wake up and energize. Coffee contains caffeine, which is a diuretic. It activates the kidneys and encourages them to push out water, increasing their energy as a result. Rubbing on your kidneys can achieve something similar but without the risks to your health. Try this sometime: avoid drinking coffee in the morning and instead rub your kidneys shortly after you wake up. Then wait about half an hour.

You may not feel as noticeably awake as when you drink coffee, but you may feel energetic enough to do what you need to do without drinking coffee.

SELF-CONFIDENCE AND ASSERTIVENESS

You may know that how people stand and hold themselves affects how they feel. If you have not known this until now, try it. Stand with poor posture and look down at the floor with a frown on your face. Stay like that for a minute. Now stand up straight, look forward, and smile. Do you notice the difference?

When people have the courage and ability to speak their minds and set healthy boundaries, it is commonly referred to as "having a backbone." Why do people say that? Why not refer to it as having big eyebrows? On some level it must be understood that having a strong, straight, healthy spine is related to saying what you feel and need to say. In the Universal Healing Tao we consider the spine to be the center of communication.

Within the Universal Healing Tao system is a series of practices called Iron Shirt Chi Kung. One of these practices is an exercise called Embracing the Tree. It is called that because when people hold this posture it looks like they are wrapping their arms around the trunk of a tree. When done properly this standing posture twists the tendons, stretches and strengthens the psoas muscles, opens the spine, and draws energy from above and below. This exercise has more steps than the ones that are outlined here, but it is worth it to learn the basics. Just from the description it is probably easy to imagine that holding this posture helps you feel strong and capable. Try the following steps to learn the posture. Go slowly and relax your body as much as possible as you successively add each step to the posture. If you tighten too much you will limit the flow of the energy and defeat the purpose of the exercise.

Note that this is a practice that should be performed only during the day. The stimulation that it creates could keep you awake at night if you practice it too late in the day or before bedtime.

Embracing the Tree

1. Stand with your feet shoulder-width apart. Bend your knees slightly. Look down and make sure your feet are both pointing straight forward. If they are not, then this will affect your entire posture. Make even contact with the ground with the bottoms of your feet. These are: 1) tips of the toes (head and brain); 2) middle of the toes (face and sinuses); 3) base of the toes (teeth, gums, and jaws); base of the pinky toe (neck); 4) outer side of the foot (arms, elbows, knees, legs); 5) inner side of the foot (neck, brain stem, thymus, spine, and bladder); 6) outer side of the ankle (lower back); 7) inner side of the ankle (lymph glands, fallopian tubes, and groin); 8) top middle area of the foot (lungs, chest, breasts, upper back); 9). Think about roots growing out of your feet and growing deep into the earth, rooting you to it and allowing energy from the earth to flow up your body through your feet.
2. Turn your knees slightly outward. Now press slightly down and outward on the ground with your heels. Your knees will naturally twist back a bit when you do that. That's fine.
3. Relax your tailbone so that your lower back flattens a bit. Then the energy can travel more easily up your spine.
4. Relax your abdomen. Breathe into your lower abdomen. Now your kua* is open.
5. Your pelvis is now curved and open. Energy can move more freely through that area.

*Your kua is the area that extends from where the front of your hip and leg and body meet to the top of your pelvis. It includes your adductor muscles, illipsoas, and hip joints.

6. Relax your chest. Let it sink in a bit.
7. Raise your arms up in front of you in a position that looks like you are hugging a tree. Leave a space the size of a ping-pong ball between the inside of your upper arms and your armpits. Your wrists should be at shoulder height. Your thumbs are pointing upward. Your fingers are spread and the fingertips on each hand are pointing at one another. There is a small space between the ends of your fingertips between your two hands.
8. Reach your arms forward a bit so that the joints in your arms open some more. Keep your shoulders relaxed. Let your scapulae relax and separate. We call this "pulling the bow."
9. Tuck your chin in slightly so that the joints in your neck open.
10. Lightly place the tip of your tongue on the roof of your mouth to close the energetic gap between the two halves of your jaws.
11. Smile. Lift up the corners of your mouth and eyes. This warms the energy and helps it to circulate.
12. Imagine that there is a thread tied to the top of your head that extends up to the North Star and attaches to it. The thread pulls up your whole body slightly like a marionette. This makes it easier for energy to flow down to your body from above.
13. Without lifting your heels or toes off of the ground, rock slowly back and forth for approximately thirty seconds or until you can feel your body tightening despite your best efforts to stay loose and relaxed.
14. Repeat this process nine times.
15. Now slowly lower your arms and rest. Notice what you feel in your arms as they come down. That is your chi. If you turn up the water pressure in a garden hose to the maximum, the hose gets stiff from the strong flow of water inside. A similar thing happens when there is strong chi flow in your arms.

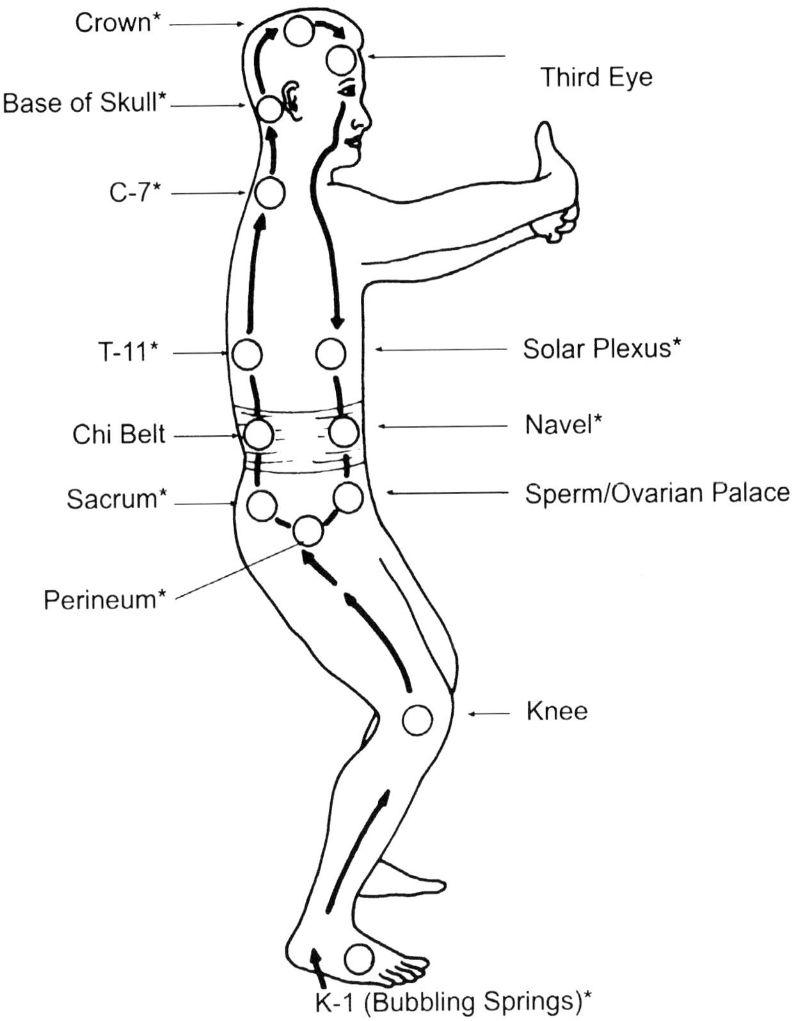

*Circle the energy nine times clockwise and nine times counterclockwise.

Fig. 7.4. Embracing the Tree, from Iron Shirt Chi Kung.

STANDING TALL

When someone is in active addiction, especially when using drugs like crack cocaine, fentanyl, or heroin, their body starts to hunch over due to the level of toxicity that has accumulated in their fascia. People in recovery often complain of feeling older than their years because their joints hurt and their body feels weak. Those effects of drug use do not have to be permanent. Fascia is the layer of connective tissue that runs throughout the body. It surrounds the tendons, ligaments, muscles, tissues, organs, nerves, bones, and joints. When the fascia is healthy and strong it is flexible and stretches as you move. When the fascia is weakened by toxic buildup, it affects all of the surrounding parts of the body. Restoring the fascia back to health is thus crucial to feeling overall wellness in the body.

The Iron Bridge

The Iron Bridge is another practice from Iron Shirt Chi Kung that will stretch your fascia and restore your posture. The practice has a yang position and a yin position. We will begin with the yang position, then go to the yin position; be sure to practice both positions.

1. Stand with your feet about one foot apart. Keep your knees straight. Point your feet straight and in line with your second toes. On each hand touch your thumb to your index finger while your arms are hanging at your sides and slightly forward. The rest of your fingers are held loosely together.
2. Breathe gently and fully into your lower abdomen. Maintain the finger positions while you reach behind you and bend your elbows back. Your palms should be facing up.
3. Arch your back. Arch from your upper and middle back, not your hips. As you arch back, tighten your thighs and buttocks and keep your knees straight.

4. Now clench your teeth and lean your head back so that you can feel a stretch in the front part of your neck. Eventually you will feel your abdomen stretch as well.
5. Exhale and return to the original standing position. Repeat three times.

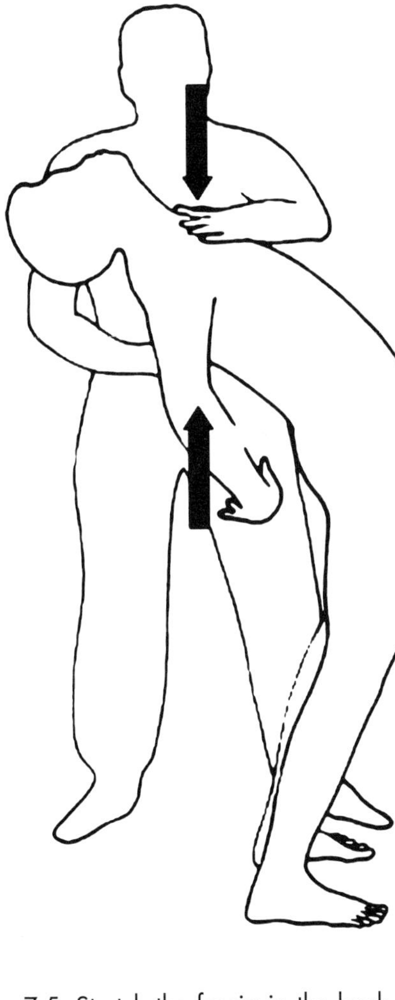

Fig. 7.5. Stretch the fascia in the back of your body by practicing the yang position of the Iron Bridge posture.

Next, the yin position of the Iron Bridge posture stretches the fascia in the back of the body.

1. Standing upright again, continue to maintain the hand position described above. This time bring your hands to the front of your body.
2. Slowly bend forward from your hip joints. Bend forward from your shoulders and chest. Round your back.
3. Let your head hang down as you descend. Your hands will eventually be near or touching the floor. Let your arms dangle.
4. Come up very slowly. You might feel dizzy at first. Slowly alternate between the yang and yang positions three times.
5. Rest.

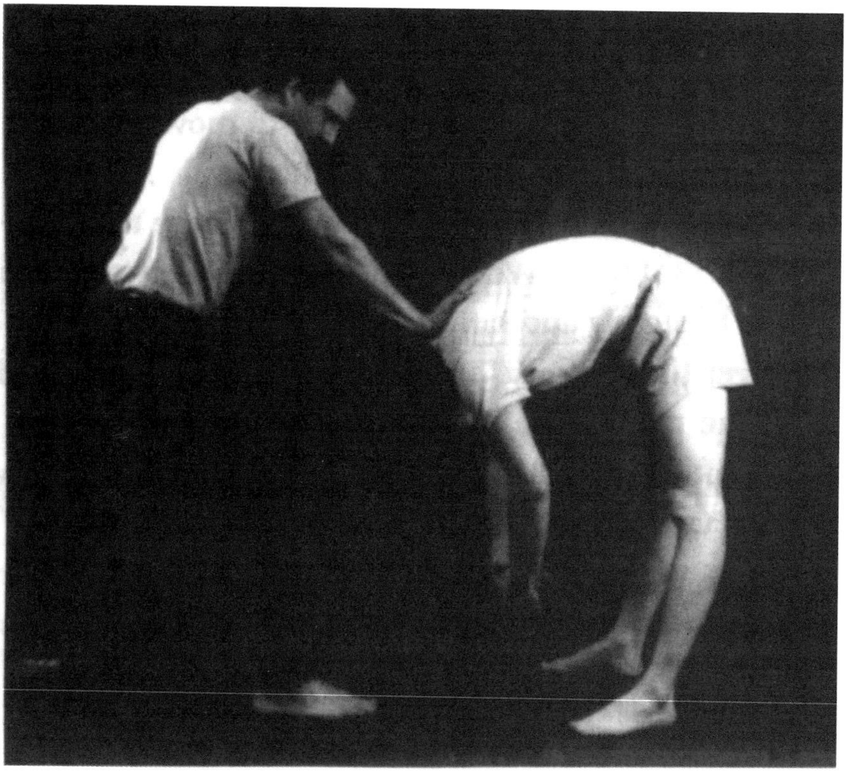

Fig. 7.6. Stretch the fascia from your groin to your neck using the Iron Bridge yin position.

ACCESSING YOUR INNATE WISDOM

Many people in recovery will refer to the "addict mind" and emphasize that it is different from the mind of a "normie," someone who does not have an addiction. It seems like the mind of someone who has an addiction is somehow viewed as less rational, more self-centered, less aware of consequences, or less wise. However, it is also important to note that those who have worked hard on their recovery and have stayed away from their addictions for many years are often regarded as being very wise. Why is this?

There are many possible explanations. One is due to the time factor: over the years, many of the cells of someone with an addiction that have been damaged will repair and heal, depression and anxiety can be treated, people can learn great life lessons in recovery, and their systems will become cleaner as toxins are released. Even after years of recovery, however, some people still feel like their minds are not as sharp and clear as they should or could be. The Wisdom Chi Kung practice can help.

Wisdom Chi Kung

Healthy energy from the internal organs can be used to energize, recharge, and nourish the mind. When the mind is empty, transformed energy from the organs can charge it with chi. To prepare for this practice, sit and rock on your sitting bones as described in chapter 5, "Preparatory Practice." Then perform the Three Minds into One Mind practice in chapter 5 to empty your upper mind into your lower mind. You are now ready to begin this practice.

1. Smile and focus on your Lower Tan Tien. Let the fire build there. Maintain 95 percent of your focus on your Lower Tan Tien while you focus your remaining attention on the other areas mentioned in this practice. Keep your heart soft.

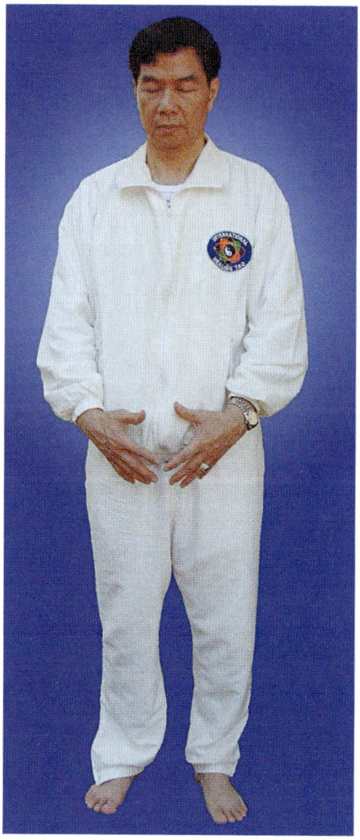

Fig. 7.7. Smile and empty your mind to your Lower Tan Tien. Let the fire build there.

2. Smile and empty your mind down to your Lower Tan Tien and your kidneys. Smile and focus on your kidneys to activate your kidney fire. Let the energy rise up from your kidneys to the back of your brain (figures 7.7 and 7.8).
3. Smile, relax, and empty your upper mind down to your bladder and sexual organs. Feel the energy build in the sexual organs and rise up to the middle of your brain (figure 7.9).
4. Smile, relax, and empty your upper mind down to your liver and gallbladder. Let them fill with chi. Allow that transformed chi to rise up to the center of the right side of your brain (figure 7.10).
5. Smile, relax, and empty your upper mind down to your heart and small intestine. Allow chi to transform those organs. Then feel that chi rise up to charge the front part of the center of your brain (figure 7.11).

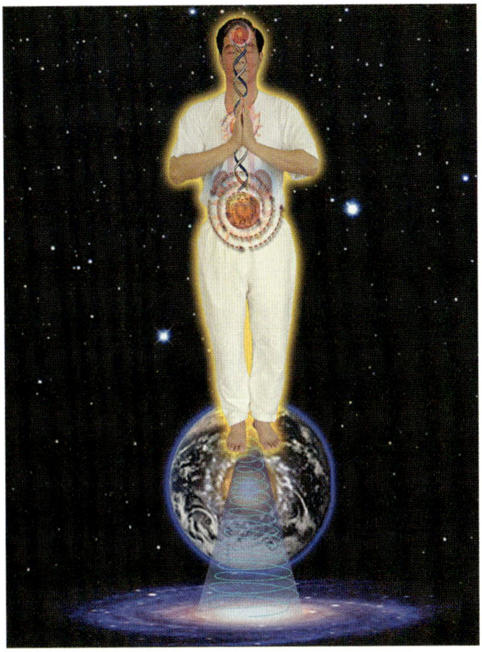

Fig. 7.8. Smile and empty your mind to your kidneys.

6. Smile, relax, and empty your upper mind down to your spleen, pancreas, and stomach. Allow the chi to transform those organs. Then feel the chi rise up to energize the left side of your brain (figure 7.12).
7. Smile, relax, and empty your upper mind down to your lungs and large intestine. Allow the chi to transform those organs. Then let the energy rise up to energize the front part of the left and right sides of your brain (figure 7.13).
8. Direct your mind down to all of your organs. When you've emptied your mind to your organs, the transformed energy from the organs can fill with chi (figure 7.14).
9. Combine that chi with good intentions and the universal cosmic energy, and that energy will be returned to you, multiplied many times over, to fill you with enhanced life force. With your brain filled with chi, be aware of a star or light above you. Maintain your awareness of your Lower Tan Tien.
10. Be aware of the universe, the stars, and the galaxies. Smile and empty your mind to the universe (figure 7.15).

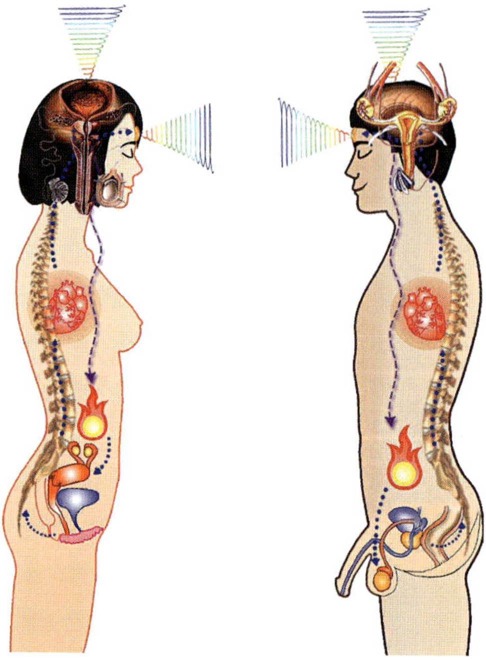

Fig. 7.9. Smile and empty your mind to your sexual organs.

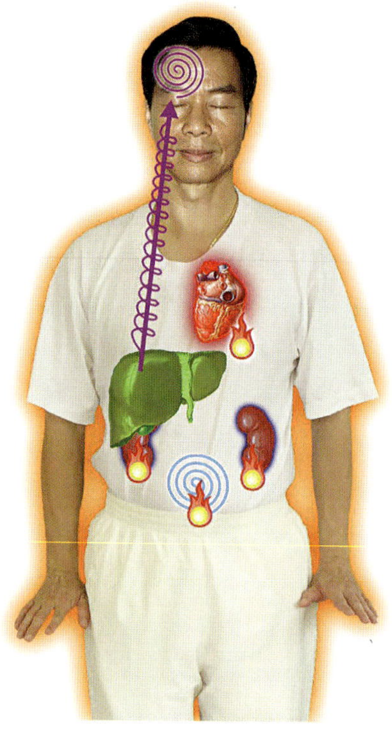

Fig. 7.10. Smile and empty your mind to your liver.

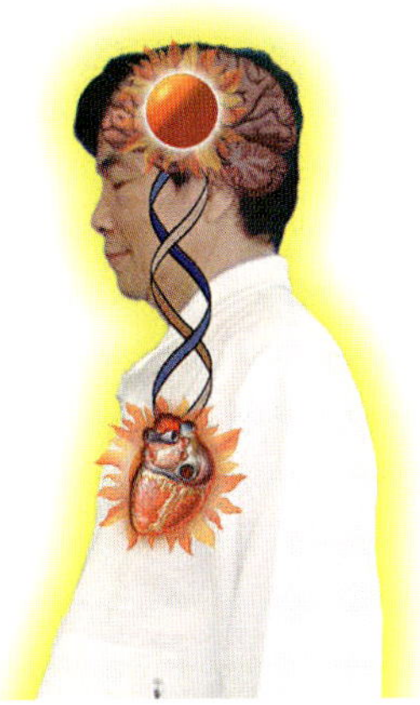

Fig. 7.11. Smile and empty your mind to your heart.

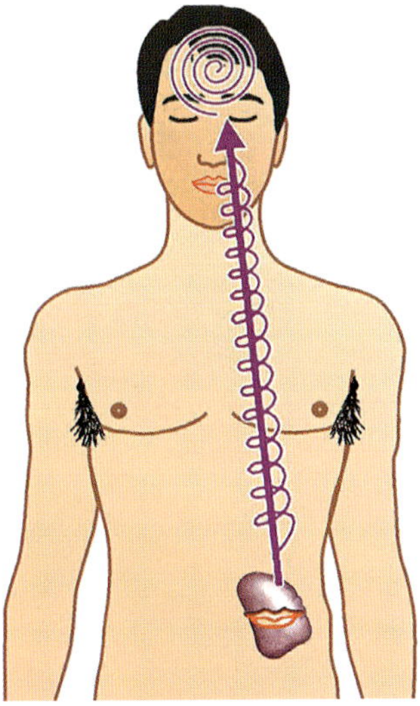

Fig. 7.12. Smile and empty your mind to your spleen.

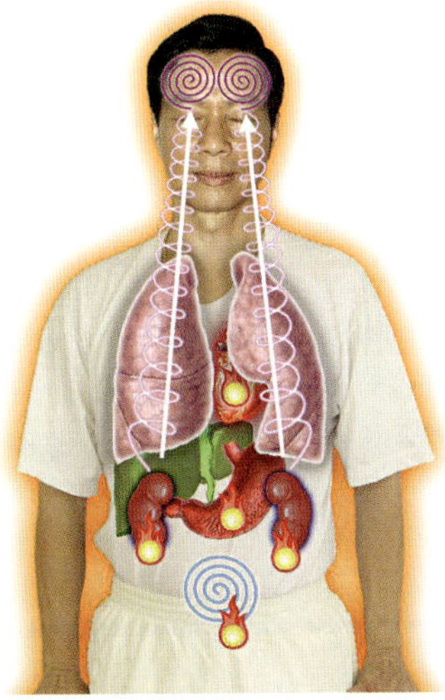

Fig. 7.13. Smile and empty your mind to your lungs.

11. Now open to receive energy from the universe. Combine the universal cosmic energy with the transformed chi in your Lower Tan Tien. The energy you shared with the universe will be returned to you many times over, to then fill your brain and your whole body (figure 7.16).
12. Hold the enhanced chi in your mind for as long as you can comfortably manage it. As your practice deepens, you will be able to hold it longer.

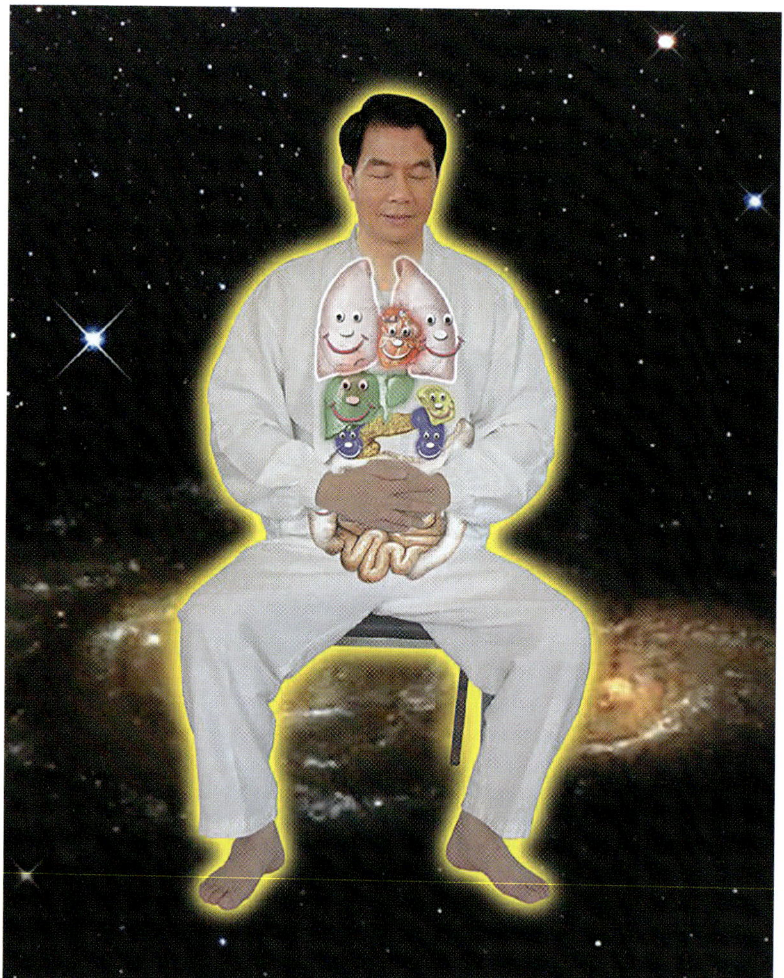

Fig. 7.14. Empty your mind so that the chi from your organs can fill it.

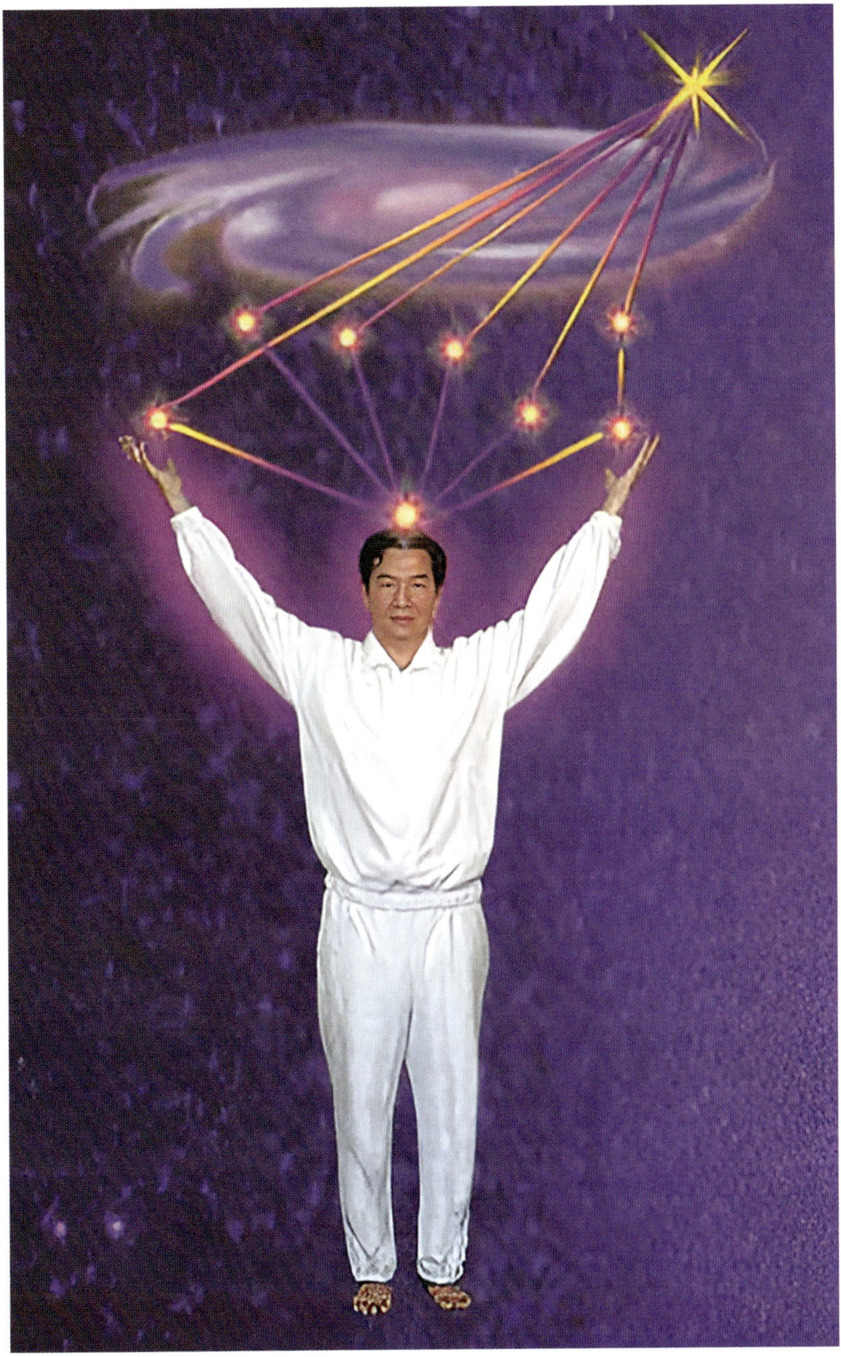

Fig. 7.15. Empty your mind to the universe.

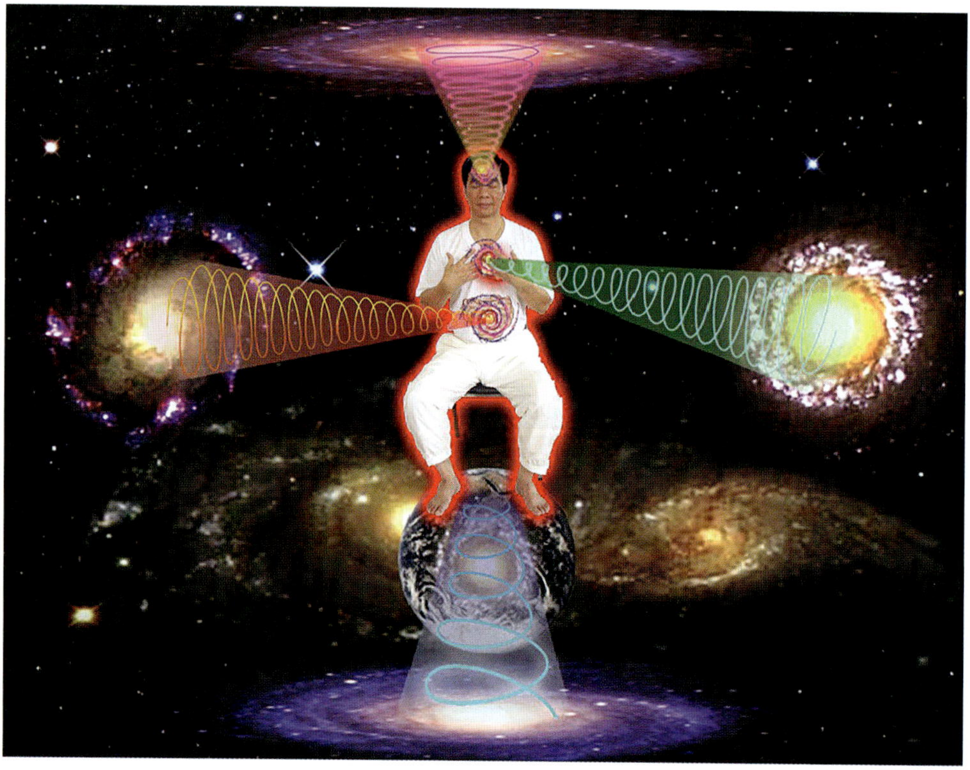

Fig. 7.16. Receive energy from the universe and blend it with the chi in your Lower Tan Tien.

13. Direct your upper mind down to your Lower Tan Tien again. Feel the enhanced energy there vibrating at a higher frequency. That enhanced chi can now flow up to energize your mind again.
14. Once your mind has filled with chi again, empty it to the universe. Once you have done this your mind will be filled with a higher force, which will increase your capacity for understanding and wisdom (figure 7.17).

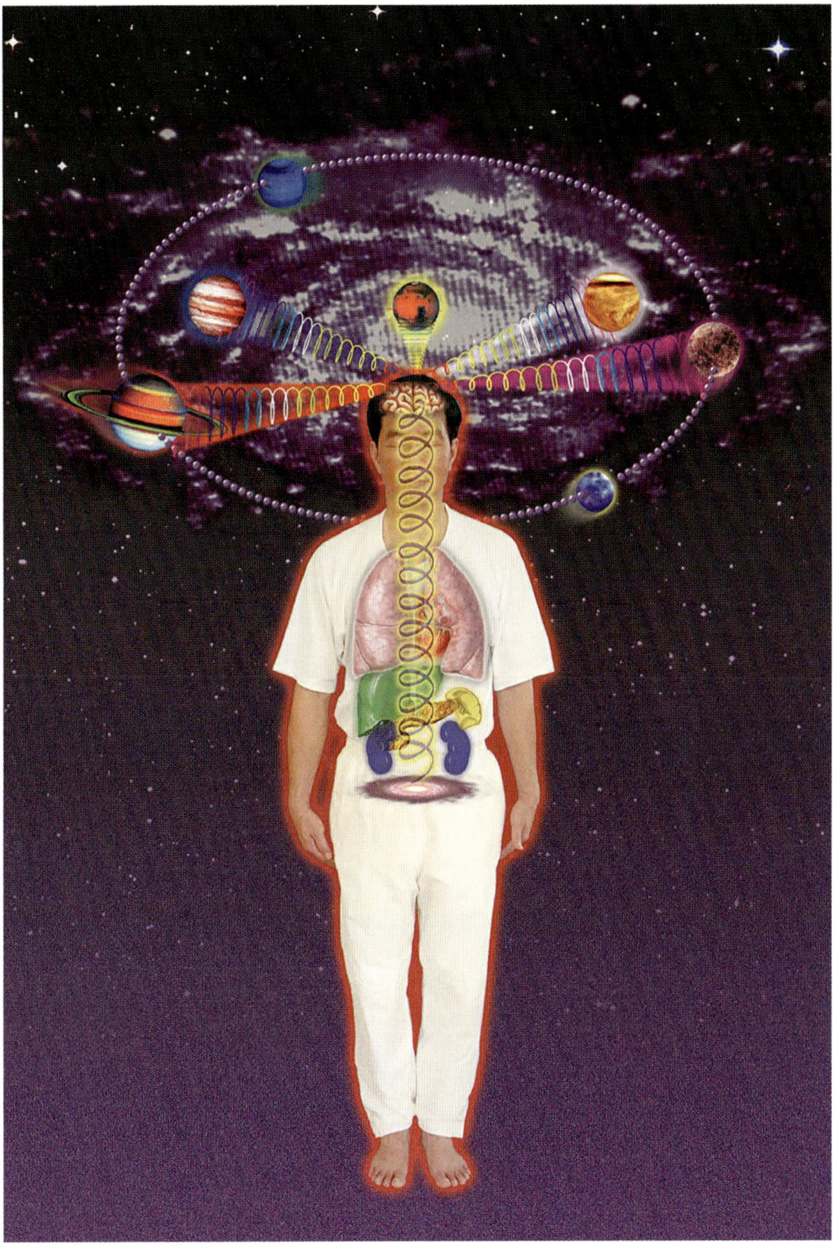

Fig. 7.17. The Wisdom Chi Kung practice uses transformed chi in your organs and the energy of the universe to energize your mind for a greater capacity for wisdom.

GATHERING SUPPORT

Recovery is a lifelong journey that typically includes many changes, and along with that, stress and confusion, so people in recovery need validation and encouragement to keep going. They may be aware that other people in their lives who do not have an addiction might judge them or not understand their experiences. At the same time, talking to people who have had to deal with an addiction does not necessarily guarantee that their advice or comments will be helpful. In fact, there is a high probability that the person dealing with an addiction will eventually have an unsatisfying interaction with someone in a support group or even with their sponsor. Some people have had bad experiences at church or with a counsellor. When they were in active addition their past dealings with untrustworthy people made it difficult for them to trust people, and so they can end up feeling let down by people when they enter recovery. Moreover, their failure to find effective support validates their belief that they cannot trust anyone.

The truth is that there are no guarantees for any of us when it comes to dealing with other people. We all have blind spots and shortcomings. What should we do, then? Should we just try to do everything on our own? That is a typical strategy, almost a rite of passage, for people in recovery—they try to handle everything themselves, only to find that they cannot. Perspective is important—how can someone in recovery see the forest for the trees when they are standing in the middle of the trees? Trying to handle everything by themselves inevitably will fail, and this is how people eventually discover that going it alone does not work—but many will try it anyway before getting true support. So it should be obvious why many people in recovery end up feeling stuck—they want support, but do not believe that effective support exists.

The solution is to change one's ideas around support. A common expression is to "take what you need and leave the rest." This means allowing yourself to decide if the feedback or advice you've received should be accepted or not. This is where paying attention to one's feelings is so important, as it's the emotional body, not the thinking mind, that decides whether something feels right. Another strategy is to be grateful that you do not operate based on the same misinformation or misconceptions that someone else seems to have. This is helpful when you're exposed to ideas that do not resonate or make sense to you. Then you do not have to categorically reject each person or support environment, and you can continue to be receptive to receiving effective support when such an opportunity presents itself.

Six Directions and Three Fires

A practice called Six Directions and Three Fires, from the Cosmic Healing branch of the Universal Healing Tao, offers a reliable source of support that you can depend on. In this practice we learn to surrender to the energy of the universe as we simultaneously open to receive energy from it. That sounds like a contradiction, but it is a state that you will eventually resonate with as you do this practice. Quantum physics has validated that time and space are merely measurements that result from our senses, not from reality. We can extend our minds to effect change far beyond what our senses can perceive and do (called *nonlocality* in quantum physics). This practice uses that concept to draw energy from the universe to us. In it we receive energetic support from the universe, so that relying on the opinions of others is not as crucial. The support you will feel comes in the form of a strong inner feeling as you draw energy from the different directions.

1. To begin, first perform the Three Minds into One Mind practice from chapter 5. This will allow you to move your focus from your head down to your energetic battery, the Lower Tan Tien (figures 7.18 and 7.19).
2. Stand with your feet together. Bend your hands outward at the wrists so that your palms face the ground and your fingers point forward. Press them down gently until your arms are slightly bent

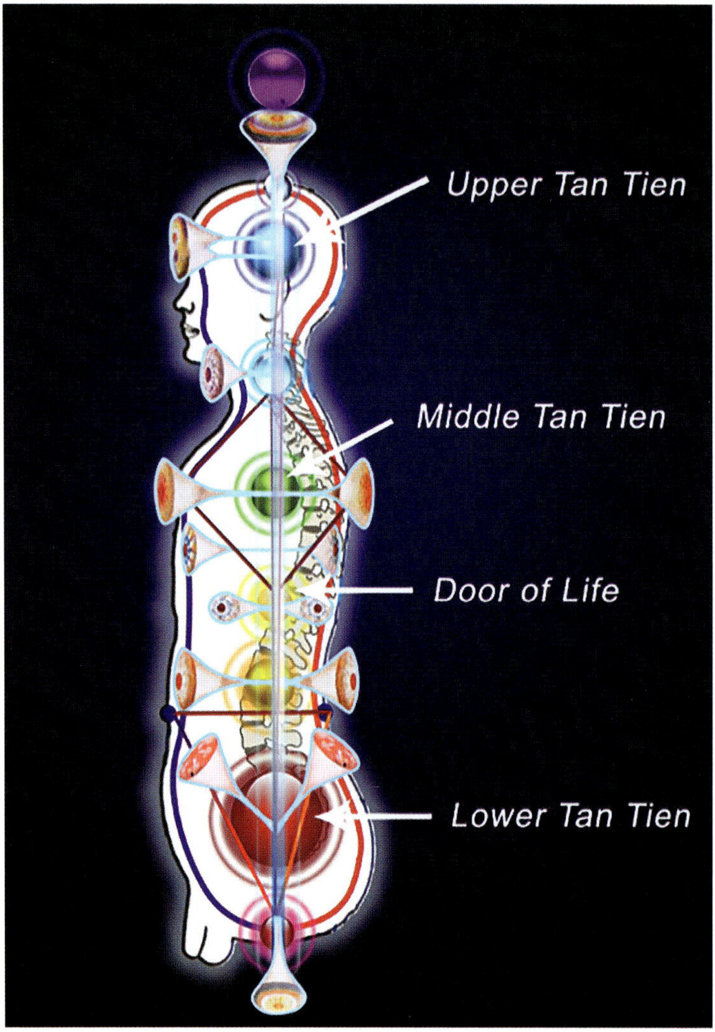

Fig. 7.18. Location of the Upper, Middle, and Lower Tan Tien.

and your palms are parallel to the ground. Contemplate the fact that you are standing on the Earth. Think about your arms and hands extending all the way down through the Earth, and to the other side of the Earth and beyond, to the universe, and beyond that, extending all the way to the primordial force. Slowly push your hands down about six inches and reach for that primordial energy.

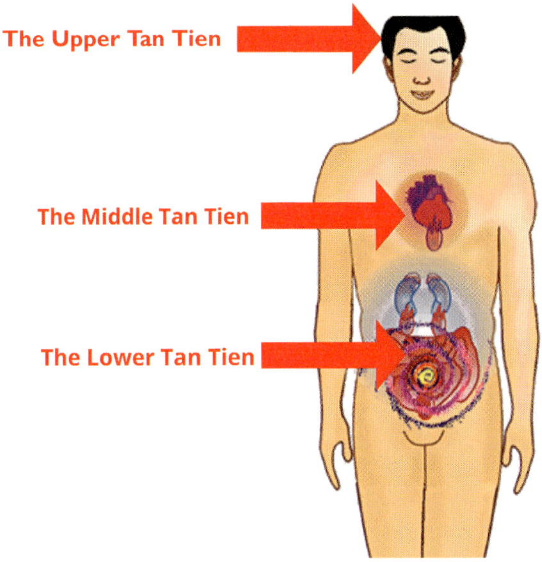

Fig. 7.19. Location of the Upper, Middle, and Lower Tan Tien.

3. Bring your hands slowly straight up about six inches on each side of your body so that your arms are slightly bent again. and visualize that you are bringing the primordial force energy with them, through your hands to your Lower Tan Tien. Think about your Lower Tan Tien filling with chi. Smile at your Lower Tan Tien.
4. Repeat this push-pull movement with your palms lowering and raising three to nine times total.
5. Visualize a small dot of light inside your Lower Tan Tien. Now visualize a big fireball in front of you. Reach forward to scoop up the energy from that fireball with your hands and then bring it back to your Lower Tan Tien. Use this fireball to light the fire in your Lower Tan Tien. Once is often enough for this part, but you can do it three times to make sure the fire is lit.
6. Feel the fire in your Lower Tan Tien burning now. This is called "fire burning under the sea." You can close your eyes to really focus on the feeling.

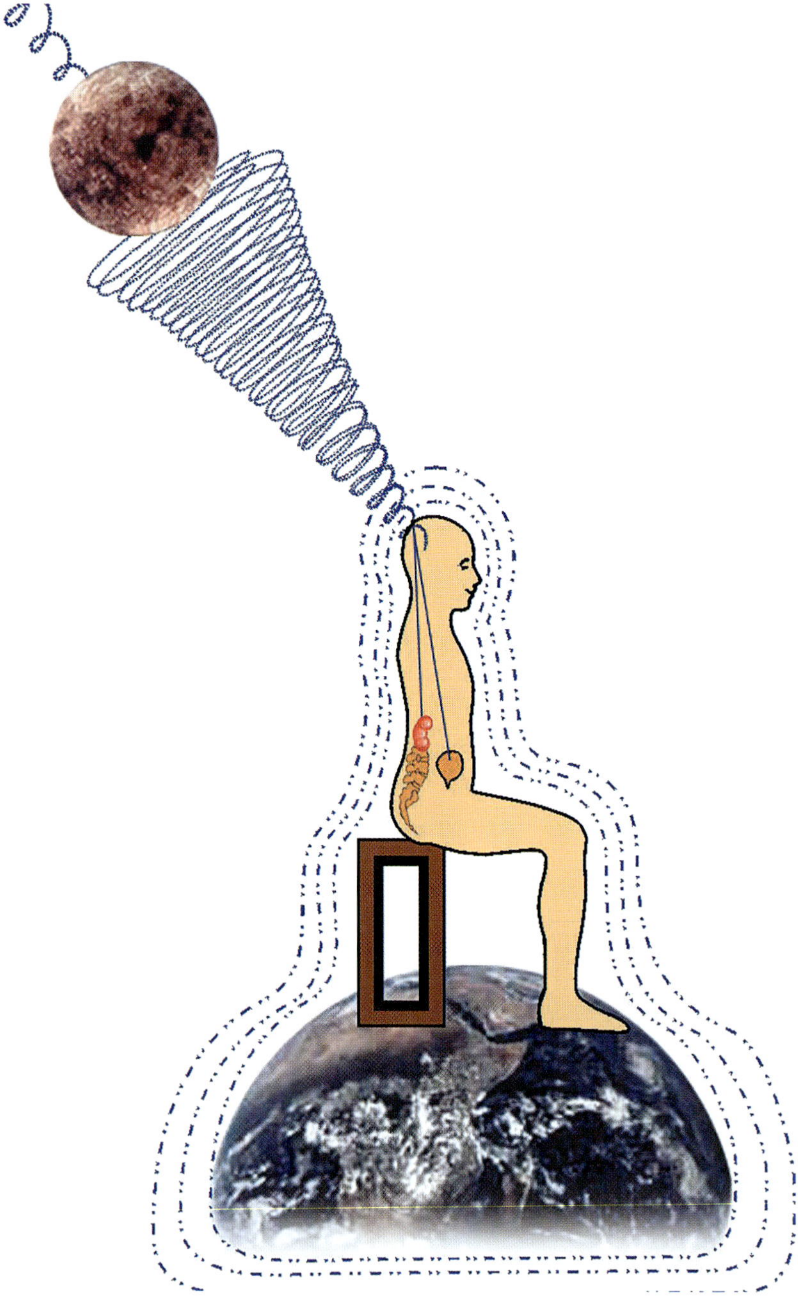

Fig. 7.20. Draw energy from the universe behind you to ignite your kidney fire.

7. Now focus on the Door of Life, located on the back directly opposite your Lower Tan Tien. Maintain your focus on your Lower Tan Tien but allow your mind to also reach out to the universe behind you (figure 7.20). Reach back with your hands and arms. See your arms growing very long so they can touch the universe behind you. Scoop up the fire from the universe and bring it back to your kidneys to activate your kidney fire. Feel that energy in your Lower Tan Tien. Feel the spiraling energy in your Tan Tien, your heart, your crown, and the universe. Repeat this motion three times.
8. Raise your elbows out to each side and reach out to each side with your palms facing upward. Feel yourself holding two fireballs there. Feel the energy from those two fireballs extending inside your body until they touch your heart with those fireballs. This activates the heart fire (figure 7.21).

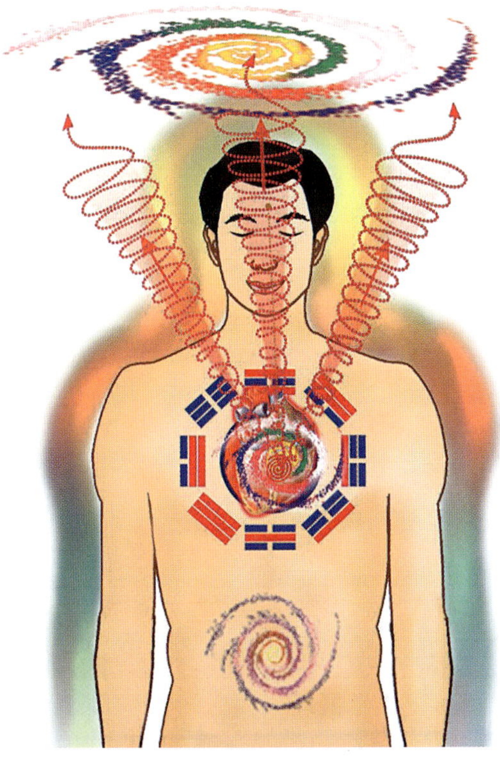

Fig. 7.21. Draw energy from the universe to activate your heart fire.

9. Allow your fingers to extend far out into the universe. Feel your Lower Tan Tien chi spiraling. Feel the energy of the universe spiraling. The universe is a type of battery charger, and you are a battery. Smile down to your heart and feel your heart soften as the universe charges more fire into you. Feel the warmth of the fire and feel the love, joy, and happiness that comes from your heart. Feel a connection to the unconditional love of the universe (figure 7.22).

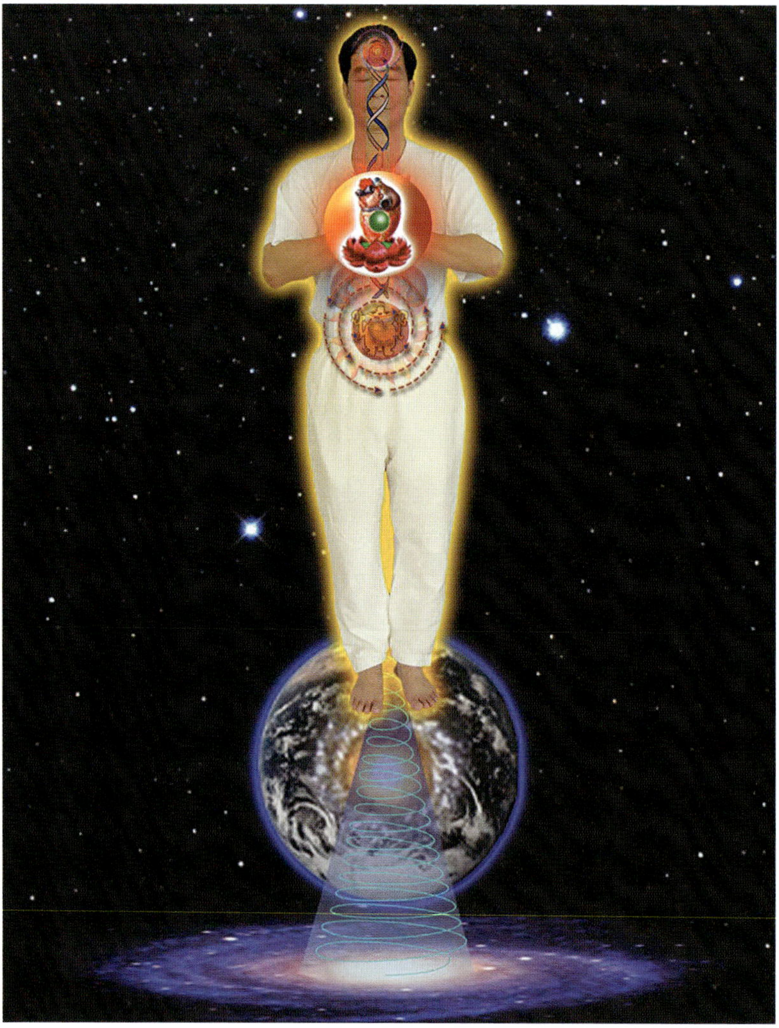

Fig. 7.22. Activate your sacred fire and circulate the energy to intensify it.

10. Bring your hands in front of your heart. Smile into your heart. Feel the fire burning there. Now connect that fire to your Lower Tan Tien fire and kidney fire to form a triangular sacred fire. Circulate the energy through this triangular fire faster and faster, up to sixty thousand revolutions per minute, to multiply the collective power of the sacred fire.
11. Now open your eyes and dim them. Smile at the universe in front of you. Reach forward with your palms. Now turn your palms inward to face you and bring energy from the universe back with your hands as your middle fingers touch your third eye. Picture a crack

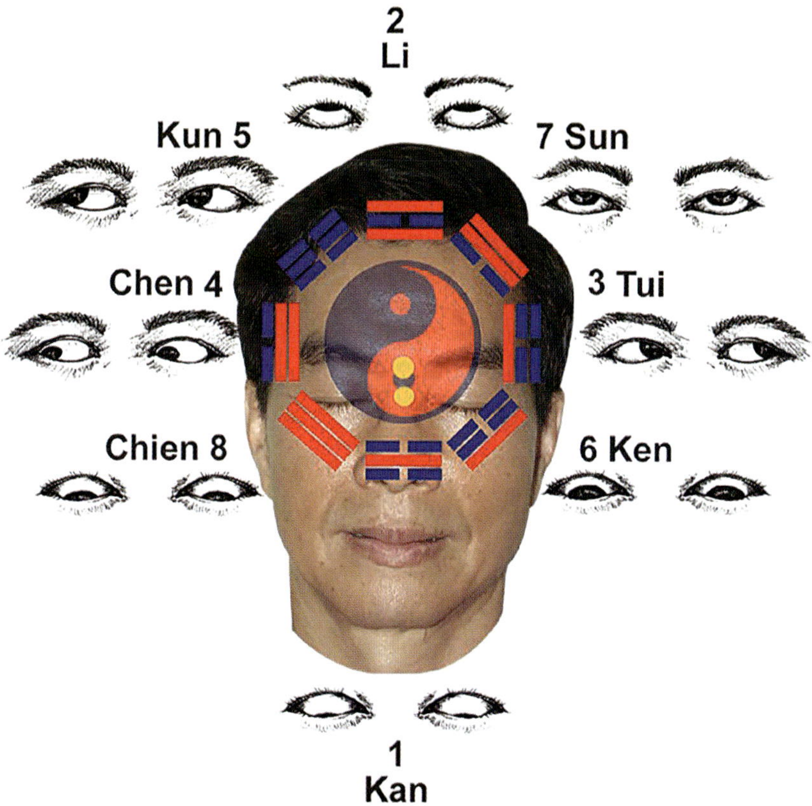

Fig. 7.23. Open your third eye.

in the middle of your forehead. Gently pull the crack open with all of your fingers. Feel the light from the heavens shining into your brain and reflecting into your organs. Open and close your third eye three to nine times (figure 7.23).

12. Now reach forward again with your palms vertical. Push and pull the universal chi to your Lower Tan Tien at least three times. You can repeat this gesture up to a hundred times (figure 7.24).
13. Move your extended hands from the front horizon to the left and right sides of your body. Your arms are slightly bent so that you can move your palms out to each side and pull them back about six inches each way while you alternate between reaching out to gather energy from the universe and then pulling it back to you. Smile and reach far out to the universe on each side. Push and pull energy from the universe on each side for three to six repetitions (figure 7.25).
14. Turn your body to the left. Turn your palms up and reach up to the universe above you. Scoop chi up from the universe above you, then turn your palms over and pour the chi over your crown. Touch your crown with all of your fingertips. Use your mind to move down the core of your body and project the chi all the way down to the perineum and down through the Earth to the universe below. Feel the chi charge your bones. Repeat this gesture until you have scooped and gathered chi three times to the left. Then turn and repeat the practice three times to the right.
15. Touch the back of your crown with all of your fingertips. Use your mind to think about pouring a waterfall of chi from your crown all the way down to the soles of your feet. Feel your fingers growing long and extending all the way down your spine to your tailbone. Focus on your three minds (head, heart, and gut), then focus on the universe and allow the universal energy to charge

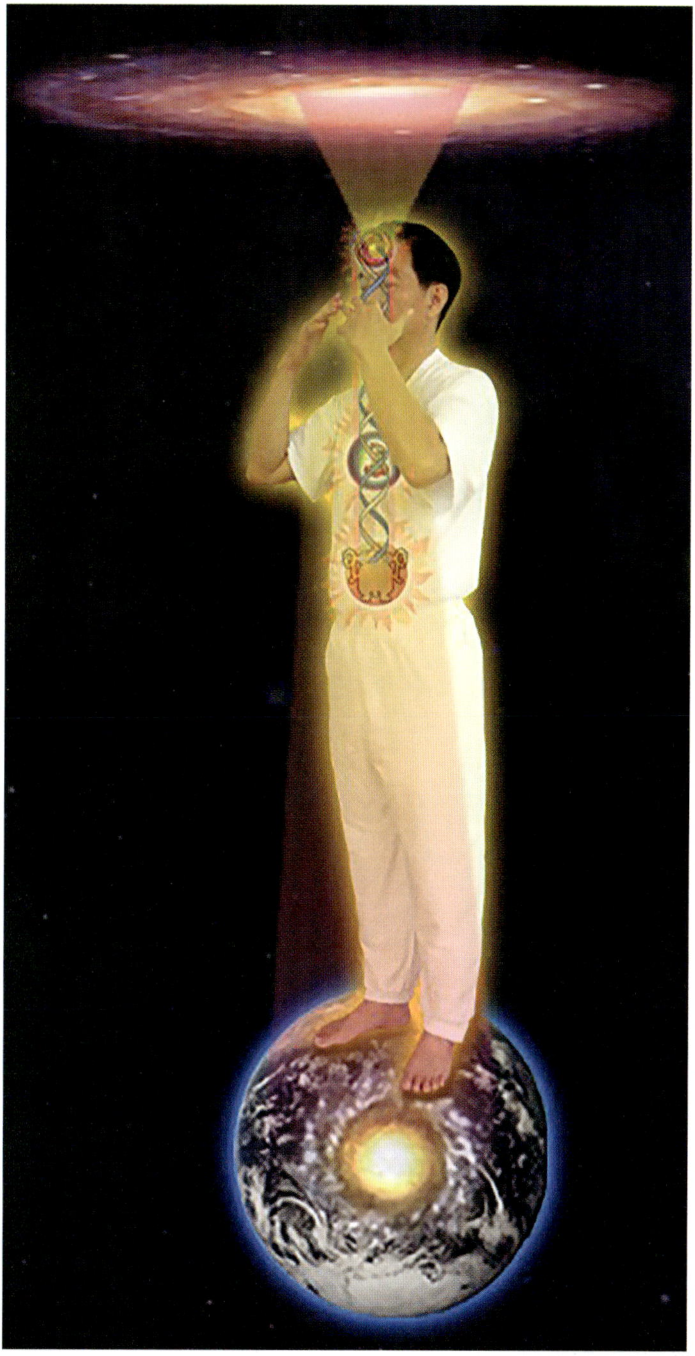

Fig. 7.24. Draw the energy from the universe in front of you.

your body. Feel the energy spiraling in your Lower Tan Tien, your heart, your crown, and in all the directions around you in the universe. Allow all the sick, negative energy in your body to leave and go down into the ground to be recycled (figures 7.26 and 7.27).

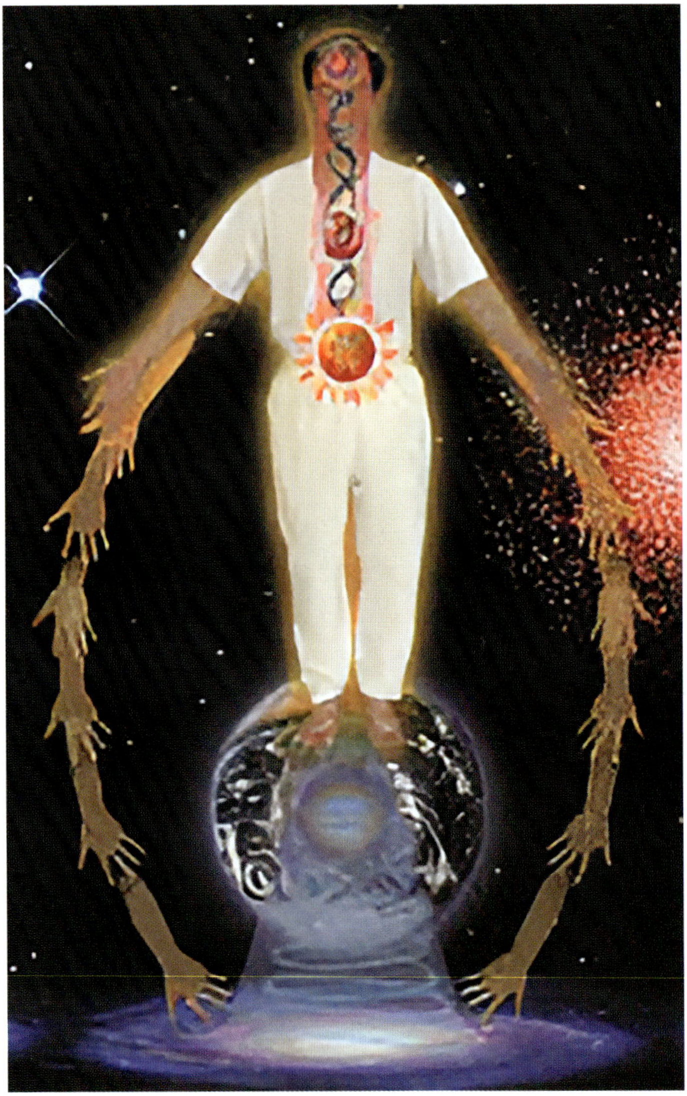

Fig. 7.25. Draw energy from the universe on your left and right sides.

16. Now move your fingers to the middle of your crown. Use your mind to think about projecting the auras of your fingers down through the middle of your body to your perineum, between your sexual organs and your anus. Focus on your perineum. Feel the chi from the universe flow into your perineum. Look for one dot of light.

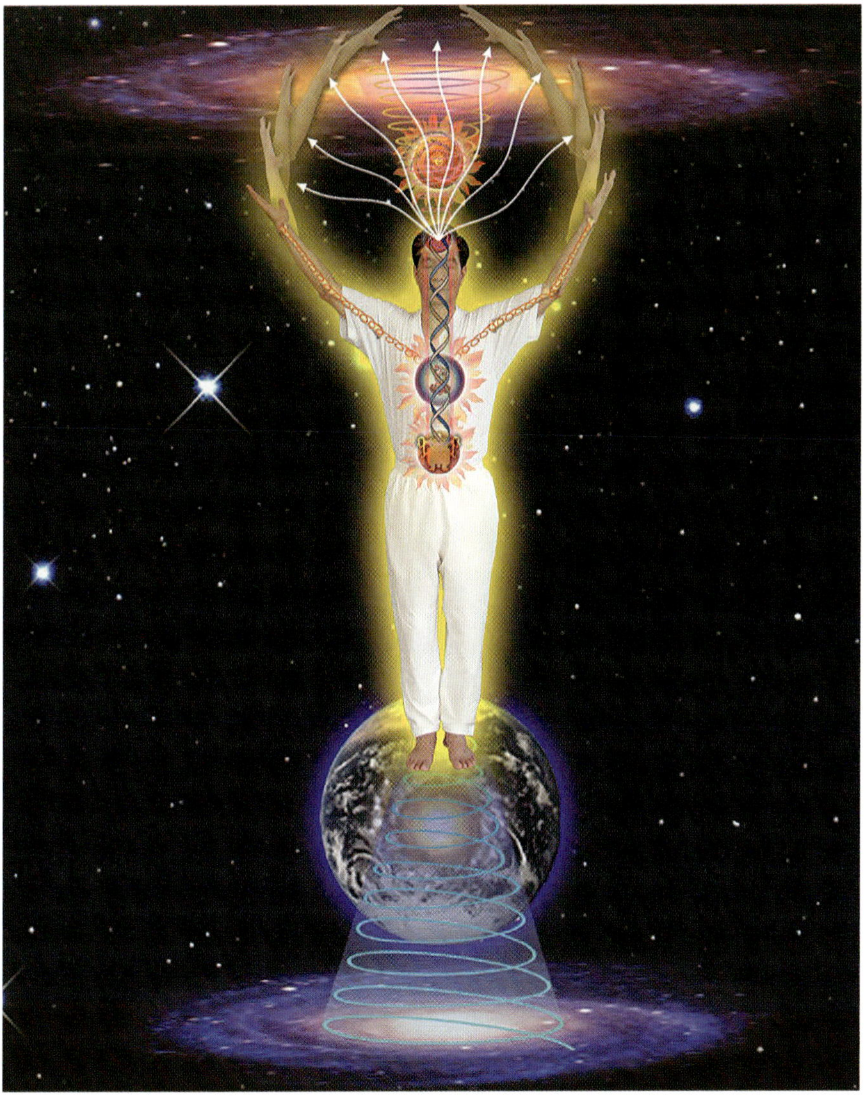

Fig. 7.26. Draw energy from the universe above you.

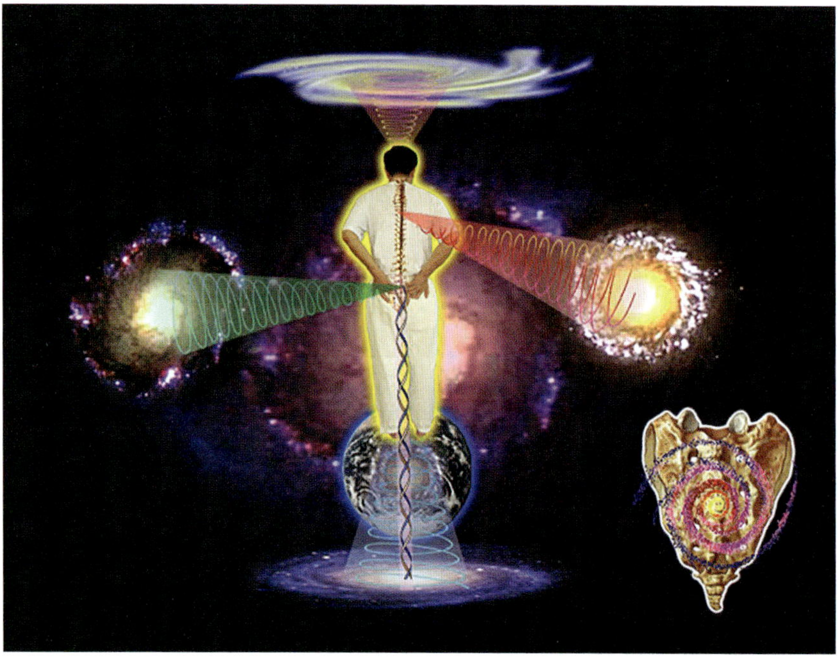

Fig. 7.27. Open your spine by pouring chi down from the back of the crown to your tailbone.

Look to the universe below and connect the energy from it to that dot of light.

17. Now you have ignited the three fires and gathered energy from the six directions. Visualize the chi as an expanding light of knowledge that radiates throughout your energy field.
18. Rest. Avoid engaging in any new activities for at least ten minutes so that the energy you have gathered can have an opportunity to cleanse and energize your energy pathways before you get caught up in the stresses of life again.

8

Practices for Transforming Toxic Patterns

Reconnecting with others in a heartfelt way and feeling the value of belonging and contributing to the people around you is an important part of recovery. Simply put, the more attached you are to healthy people and activities, the less you will be pulled to people and activities that are unhealthy. The more time you have in recovery, the more you will naturally crave a healthier and more meaningful life. But knowing how to cultivate healthy habits and a heartfelt sense of connection with others when there hasn't been much experience of that is another matter altogether.

INCREASING COMPASSION

The Inner Smile practice provides a way to transform negative energy in each of the yin organs so they can produce the positive qualities of each organ, known as their "virtues." Gathering and combining the virtues of each organ in the natural order of energy flow in the body, as we do in this practice, will increase compassion (figure 8.1).

Positive Emotions Creation Cycle
The growing alchemical cycle of the five elements

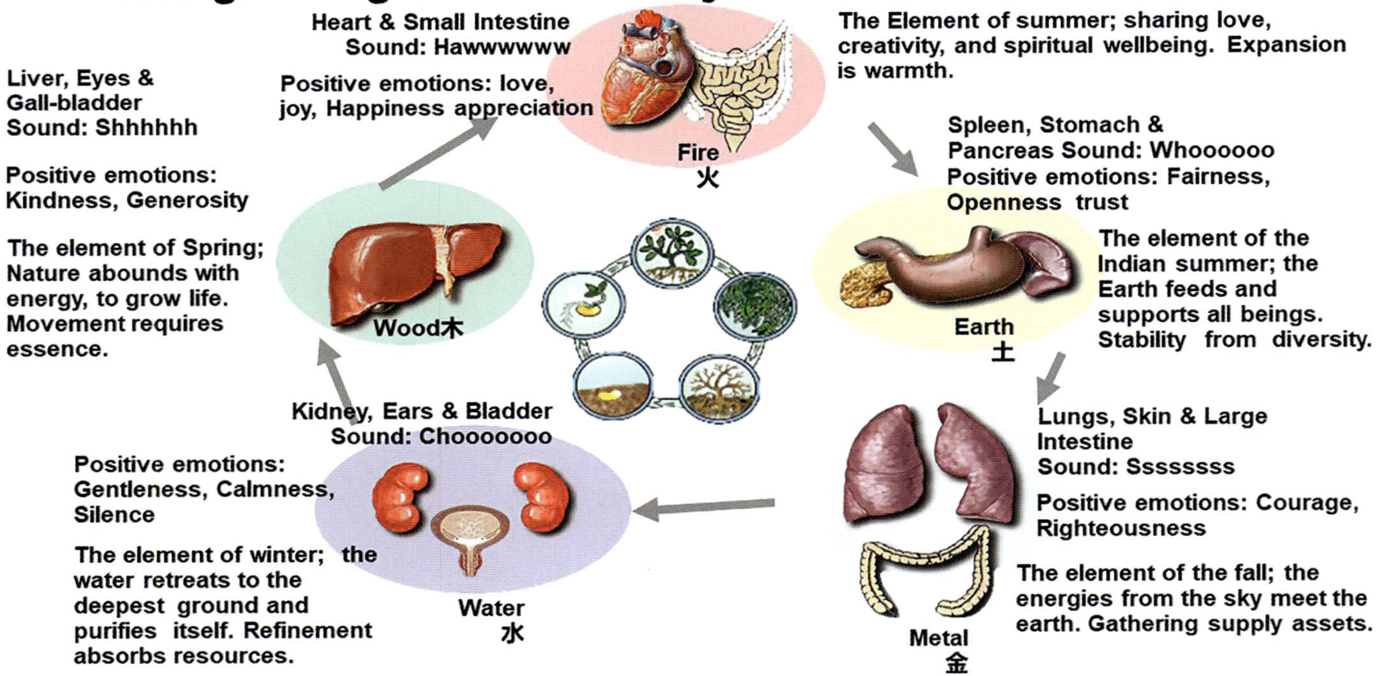

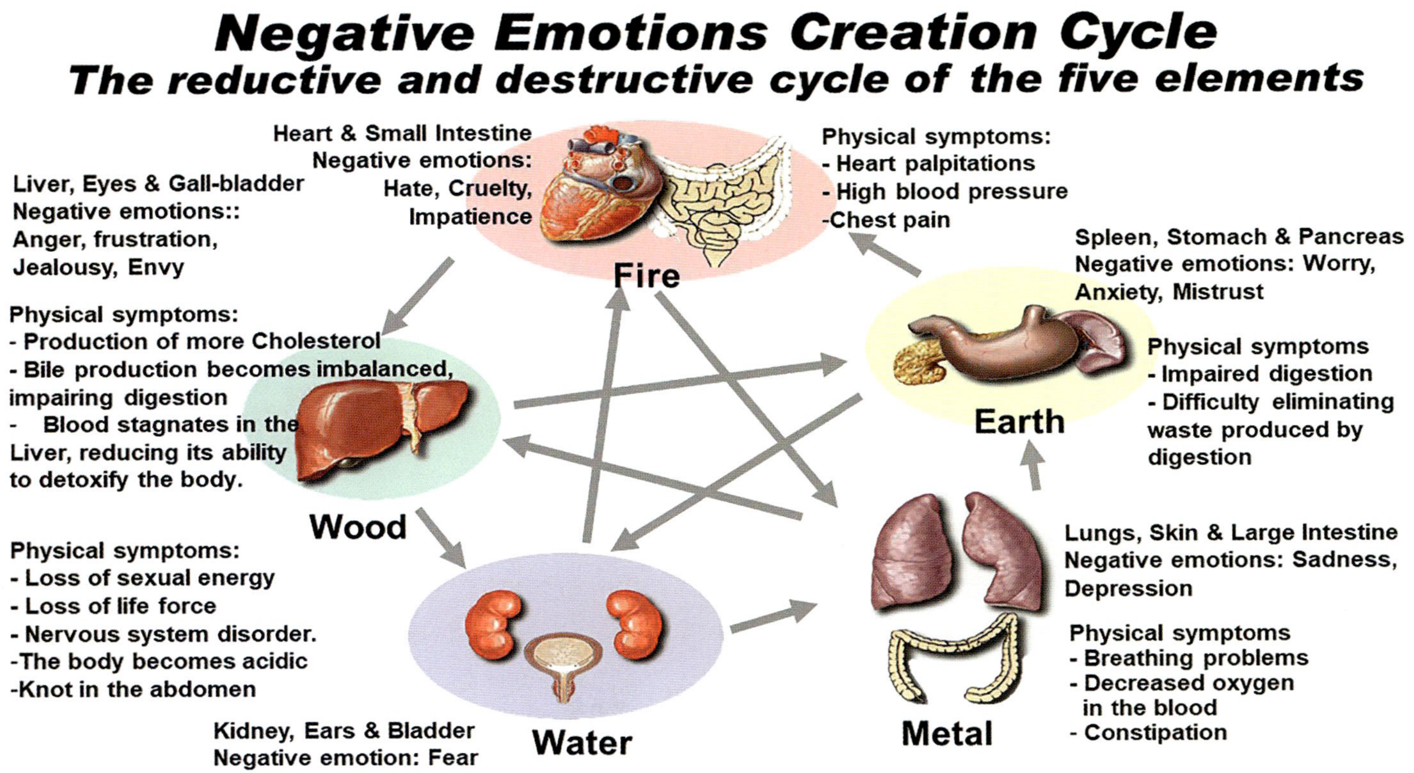

Fig. 8.1. Positive and negative emotions can be produced by each organ depending on how we feed them.

The Inner Smile also addresses many of the tendencies, habits, and emotions that can lead to or keep one in active addiction. Those emotions and habits are called "defects of character" in the language of the 12 Steps; Taoists delineate them as follows:

- The negative emotions that can be produced by the heart are hastiness, impatience, hatred, and cruelty. The Inner Smile practice can transform those emotions into the virtues of joy, love (including self-love), and happiness.
- The negative states that are produced by the spleen are worry, negative thinking, and overthinking. The Inner Smile transforms them into the virtues of openness and trust.
- The Inner Smile transforms grief, sadness, loss, and depression in the lungs into courage and righteousness.
- The kidneys can produce fear, stress, guilt and anxiety. The Inner Smile can transform them into calmness, gentleness, and stillness.
- A lack of creativity and vitality is produced when the sexual organs are toxic and unbalanced. The Inner Smile transforms them to restore their inherent creativity and vitality.
- The liver can produce anger, frustration, jealousy, envy, and resentment. Practicing the Inner Smile provides a way to transform those emotions to the virtues of the liver, which are generosity and kindness.

Note that this practice does not treat negative emotions and states as something to be avoided. Their energetic content, even when negative, provides the needed raw material that can be transformed into healthier and more useful qualities.

The Inner Smile

The Inner Smile is connected to another practice that will be described later in this chapter, the Microcosmic Orbit, a practice that promotes the healthy circulation of energy to all the organs of the body. Both practices work with the energy that flows through the Functional and Governor vessels of the body. The Governor Vessel ascends up the back of the body from the coccyx to the head, then down the front of the body to the space between the nose and the upper lip; the Functional Vessel (also known as the Conception Vessel) flows between the perineum and the space between the chin and the lower lip. They connect to form an elliptical orbit. The points along those two channels connect to important acupuncture points in the body. Both vessels are addressed in the Inner Smile practice. We will focus on the Functional Vessel first, then the Governor Vessel (figure 8.2).

1. Sit on the edge of a chair with your eyes closed and your hands clasped together. Your feet are flat on the floor.

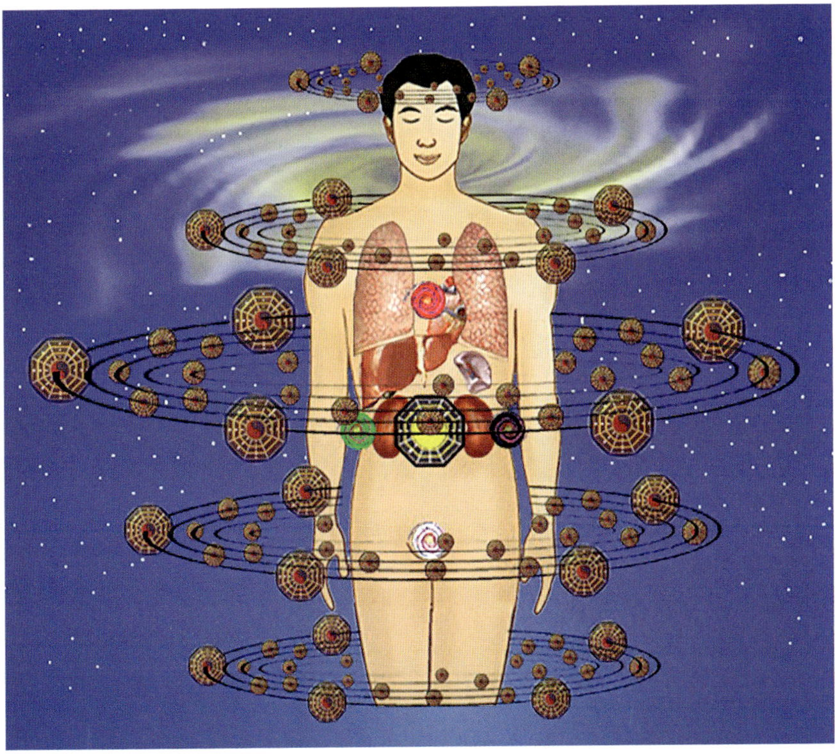

Fig. 8.2. The Functional and Governor vessels of the body.

2. Focus on the smiling energy in front of you. Breathe it into your eyes. Let that smiling energy enter the point between your eyebrows. Let it flow from there to your nose and cheeks. Let it lift up the corners of your eyes and mouth (figure 8.3).
3. Lift the tip of your tongue up so that it rests on your upper palate just behind your front teeth. Smile down from your nose and cheeks to your neck and throat, to your thyroid, parathyroid, and thymus glands. Smile at your heart and allow the virtues of your heart to spread feelings of love and joy to your spleen, lungs, kidneys, genitals, and liver.

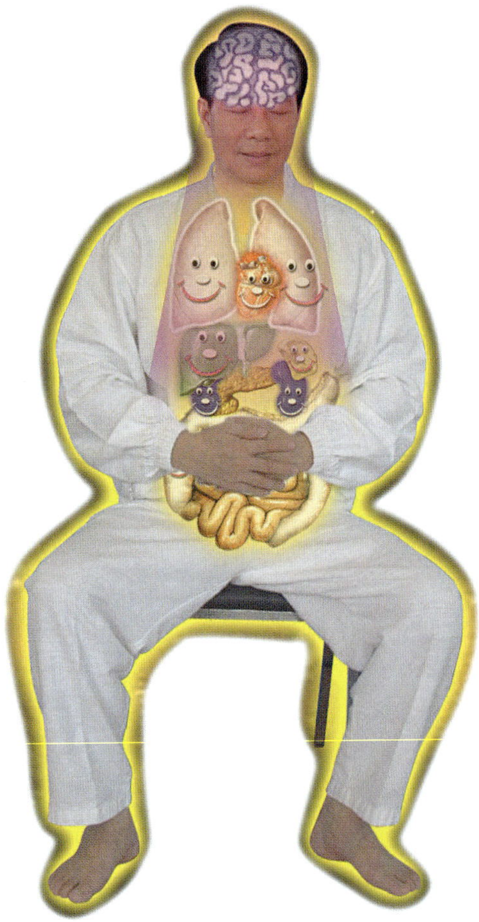

Fig. 8.3. Front line of the Inner Smile practice.

The next steps in this meditation focus on the middle line of the body, which rules the digestive tract (figure 8.4):

4. Bring your smiling energy back to your eyes. Now allow that energy to travel down to your mouth. Run your tongue along the outside gum line of your top and bottom teeth until you have a mouthful of saliva. Now swish it in your mouth like mouthwash but do not swallow it yet. Open your mouth and "chew" the air loudly to oxygenate the saliva.
5. Now close your mouth, exhale, and forcefully swallow the saliva to push it down into your body. Smile down to your stomach, small intestine (the duodenum, jejunum, and ileum), large intestine (ascending colon, transverse colon, and descending colon), rectum, and anus.

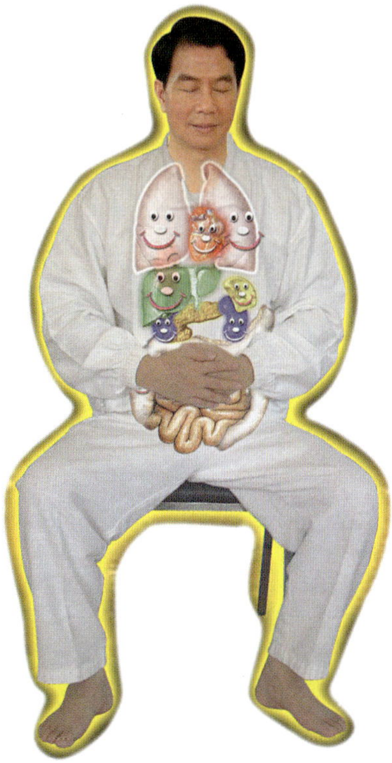

Fig. 8.4. Middle line of the Inner Smile practice.

The last part of this meditation focuses on the back line of the body, the Governor Vessel (figure 8.5):

6. Smile and focus on the mid-eyebrow point and the pituitary gland behind it. Direct that smiling energy back toward the inside of your brain, to what is called the third room, which is the small cavity deep in the center of your brain. Smile at your thalamus gland and then your pineal gland (which Taoists call the Crystal Palace). Then smile at the left and right sides of your brain.
7. Smile at your midbrain and brain stem and at the base of your skull (called the Jade Pillow). Smile down at your seven cervical vertebrae, twelve thoracic vertebrae, five lumbar vertebrae, sacrum, and tailbone.
8. Bring your smiling energy back to your eyes. Smile down at each of the three lines in succession. Now smile down at all of them at once, feeling bathed in a cooling waterfall or glowing sunshine of cosmic energy, smiles, joy, and love. Notice how you feel warm and connected to yourself and the world around you.

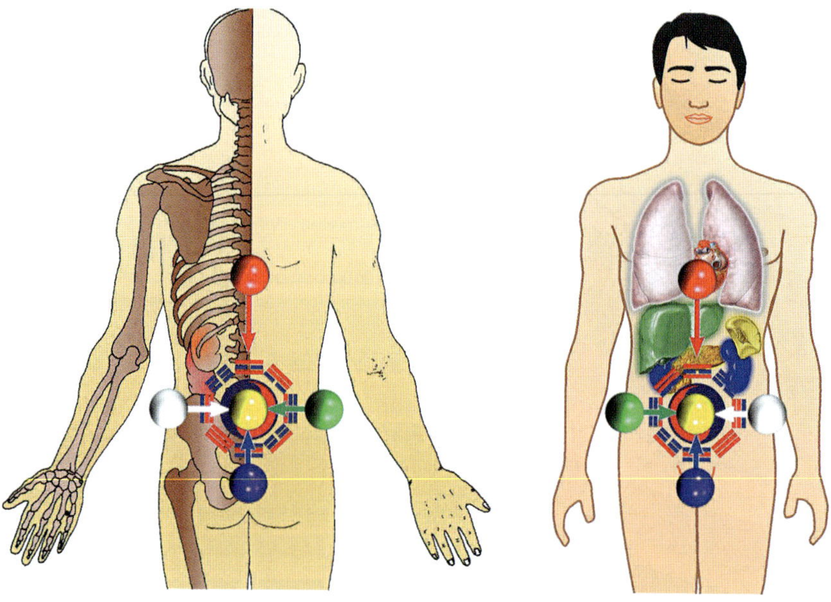

Fig. 8.5. Back line of the Inner Smile practice.

This practice is a practical way to make sure that you are following the "self first" dictum that is encouraged in recovery. The concept is similar to how people treat their vehicles. It's important to make sure that you have enough fuel in your car so that it will continue to run. People are the same—we need enough chi to function and keep going.

When we practice the Inner Smile regularly, we feel better, and those around us can sense it. Then other people will be more drawn to us and more comfortable around us. In everyday discourse we say things like "She has a magnetic personality" and "I get a good hit off of him." On some level we know that we can sense the energy of others. Sometimes people lament that recovery is not providing them with the enjoyment they want. If they do not understand what's missing—compassion for oneself and for others—they tend to want to blame other people and situations. Sometimes they even blame their Higher Power. Often they are unknowingly driving away people who could help them have a more enjoyable life because they have not yet discovered how to transform their negative energy. This practice is such a transformer.

DISSOLVING URGES

The urge to use something addictive occurs when the chi in the body is stagnant. When this happens, the body automatically demands something powerful to get energy. When someone has a history of using something addictive, their body remembers how that substance helped them feel better at least temporarily, and so they are drawn to that addictive substance or activity when their chi is not circulating properly. The Microcosmic Orbit practice addresses this. It is a natural way to open the channels and get chi to flow properly without having to resort to something addictive.

The Microcosmic Orbit

The Microcosmic Orbit is a foundational practice of the Universal Healing Tao. It involves awakening, circulating, and directing chi through the two major energy channels of the body, the Governor Vessel and the Functional Vessel. When you practice this meditation regularly, you will eventually notice that your thinking is less impulsive, you will second-guess yourself less, and your emotions will be much more manageable. This seems to happen because your energy is much more evenly distributed throughout the whole body, which is precisely the point of this exercise. The Microcosmic Orbit eliminates stress and nervous tension, energizes the internal organs, restores health to damaged tissues, and builds a strong sense of well-being. It strengthens the original chi and teaches us how to circulate it. It opens the locations in the body where energy can be absorbed, condensed, and transformed into fresh chi. The main acupuncture points and meridians are connected to the orbit, and circulating chi through the orbit feeds those channels.

The main points of the Microcosmic Orbit are:

1. **Navel:** The navel is our first connection to the outside world through which we received nutrition and oxygen while in utero. This area retains its energetic significance throughout life. The navel is the point for centering and connection to all the organs. It is also the entrance to the Lower Tan Tien cauldron, which is the place where we gather, transform, and store energy.
2. **Sexual center:** In men this is called the Sperm Palace, which starts at the base of the penis. In women it's called the Ovarian Palace and is located above the pubic bone. To find the Ovarian Palace, place your thumbs on your navel and make the index fingers come together below. Where two index fingers meet is the location of the Ovarian Palace. The area where the pinkie fingers naturally touch is where ovaries are located. Sexual energy is the only energy that can be transformed into the life force and multiplied. When this energy is not used for procreation, it is easily lost through excessive sexual activity.

3. **Perineum:** Located between the anus and the sexual organ, the perineum, known as the Gate of Life and Death, is a very important point connected to the pelvic floor. If the pelvic floor is weak, this point is where the life force may leak out. If the pelvic floor is strong, a person can use the muscle of the pelvic floor to draw energy into the body. The perineum has a close connection to earth energy. When this point is open, the person feels grounded and secure. If it is blocked, the person feels insecure and unsure.
4. **Sacrum:** The sacrum is a pump that moves spinal fluid to the brain. Moving the base of the spine and using the mind to move energy up the spine helps keep the brain young and vibrant. The sacrum is connected to the earth force, the original force, so activating its energy can increase one's life force and vibrancy.
5. **Kidney center:** This center, known as the Door of Life, is located on the spine opposite the navel and is connected to our prenatal energy, which is the original chi. When people live in stress and fear they deplete this energy, and this weakens the entire body.
6. **Adrenal gland center:** This center is located on the spine opposite the solar plexus center. It controlled by the adrenal glands and is very sensitive to stress. Its energy can be quickly drained by stimulants and drugs. When the adrenal center is open, life feels easy and free. When it is closed, life is difficult and blocked.
7. **Center opposite the heart:** This center is located on the spine opposite the heart center. It can contribute to creating the heart's radiance and shining. When this center is open, its energy protects the heart and the person experiences feelings of freedom, hope, and purpose. When it is blocked, the person will tend to feel melancholy, blocked, confused, and weighed down.
8. **Point opposite the throat:** This point is easy to find by locating the big protruding vertebra at the base of the neck, cervical vertebra 7 (C7). This point connects energy from the body to energy in the higher energy centers in the brain. If this point is blocked, people

often feel inadequate and restricted in their expressions. When it is open, it is easier to connect with other people with compassion.

9. **Small brain point, or Jade Pillow:** This point is located above the last cervical vertebra at the base of the skull. It is connected to breathing, and when it is open it helps us receive insights from the universe. This point is connected to the crown and third eye and stores yin energy. If this point is open but not connected to other points, too much energy can enter the brain, causing delusions and pressure. Opening the Microcosmic Orbit prevents this and ensures an even distribution of energy.
10. **Crown:** The crown point, or Crystal Palace, is located at the top of the head. To find this point, draw a line connecting the tips of the ears and going through the highest point of the head, and another line starting from the point between the two eyebrows all the way down to the base of the skull. This is an important energy point of connection to the forces of the universe. When the Crystal Palace is activated, it illuminates the entire head, providing clarity, inner guidance, and insights. If it is blocked, it can lead to delusions, confusion, and lack of direction (figure 8.6).

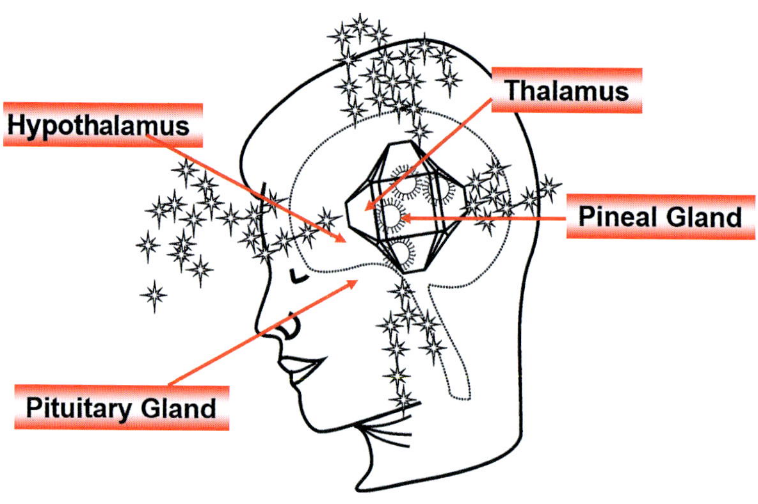

Fig. 8.6. The crown point and the Crystal Palace, which includes the pineal gland, pituitary gland, thalamus, and hypothalamus.

11. **Mid-eyebrow point:** This point is energetically connected to the middle of the forehead, the point between the two eyebrows, at the top of the nose. It connects us to higher wisdom and universal light.
12. **Heavenly Pool:** This is the point located on the roof of the mouth. When you place the tip of your tongue there, the two channels, yin and yang, become one orbit. There are three positions of the tongue: the wind position, located behind the front teeth; the fire position, which connects to the heart energy and is located further back on the palate; and the water position at the back. Usually, in the beginning it is easier to start with the wind position.
13. **Throat point:** This point is located in the V-shaped space between two collarbones. It is connected to speech and communication. In Taoist philosophy, the tongue is a sense organ of the heart, so the throat point, located halfway between the ears and the tongue, serves as an important energy bridge between the two. When this point is open, it is easier to express yourself with clarity and confidence. When it is closed, expression and communication become more difficult.
14. **Heart center:** The heart energy center on the Microcosmic Orbit is located on a direct line between the navel and the throat center, one inch above the tip of the sternum. The heart center can be opened with love, joy, and happiness. The heart center creates radiance, beauty, and a connection to universal love.
15. **Solar plexus center:** The solar plexus center is located halfway between the heart center and the navel. It is connected to the spleen, pancreas, stomach, and liver. A strong solar plexus deters negative emotions and radiates a strong aura, like a little sun. This center can be strengthened by imagining sunshine radiating from this point. When it is open, the person feels daring and bold, and when it is closed, the person may be more fearful and unsure.
16. **Point under the knees:** This point can store additional spiritual energy.

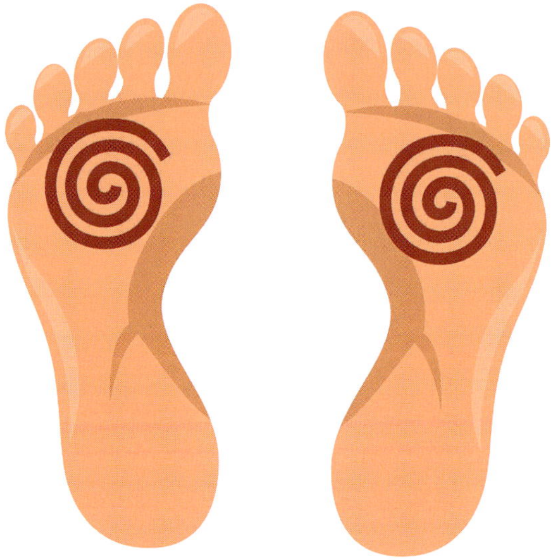

Fig. 8.7. Bubbling Springs point.

17. **Bubbling Springs point:** This point is located on the soles of both feet, in the soft spot or depression on the sole. This point can draw in the earth force and is important for practicing grounding and stability (figure 8.7).
18. **Big toe:** This point is on the lateral side of each big toe and it helps balance spiritual energy.
19. **Kneecap:** This point is in the middle of the upper portion of both knees. It helps refine earth energy as it goes up the legs.

1. Sit on the edge of a chair. Smile and focus on your Lower Tan Tien, located at the intersection between your navel, kidneys, and sexual organs, where your original chi is stored. Feel the pulsing there. Notice how it feels. It may feel tense or relaxed, cool or warm, contracted or expansive. The more you smile and focus on it, the more you will feel the tingling, warm, expansive, pulsing, electric, or magnetic sensations of healthy chi. Allow that chi to grow and expand. Then let it flow out to your navel center.

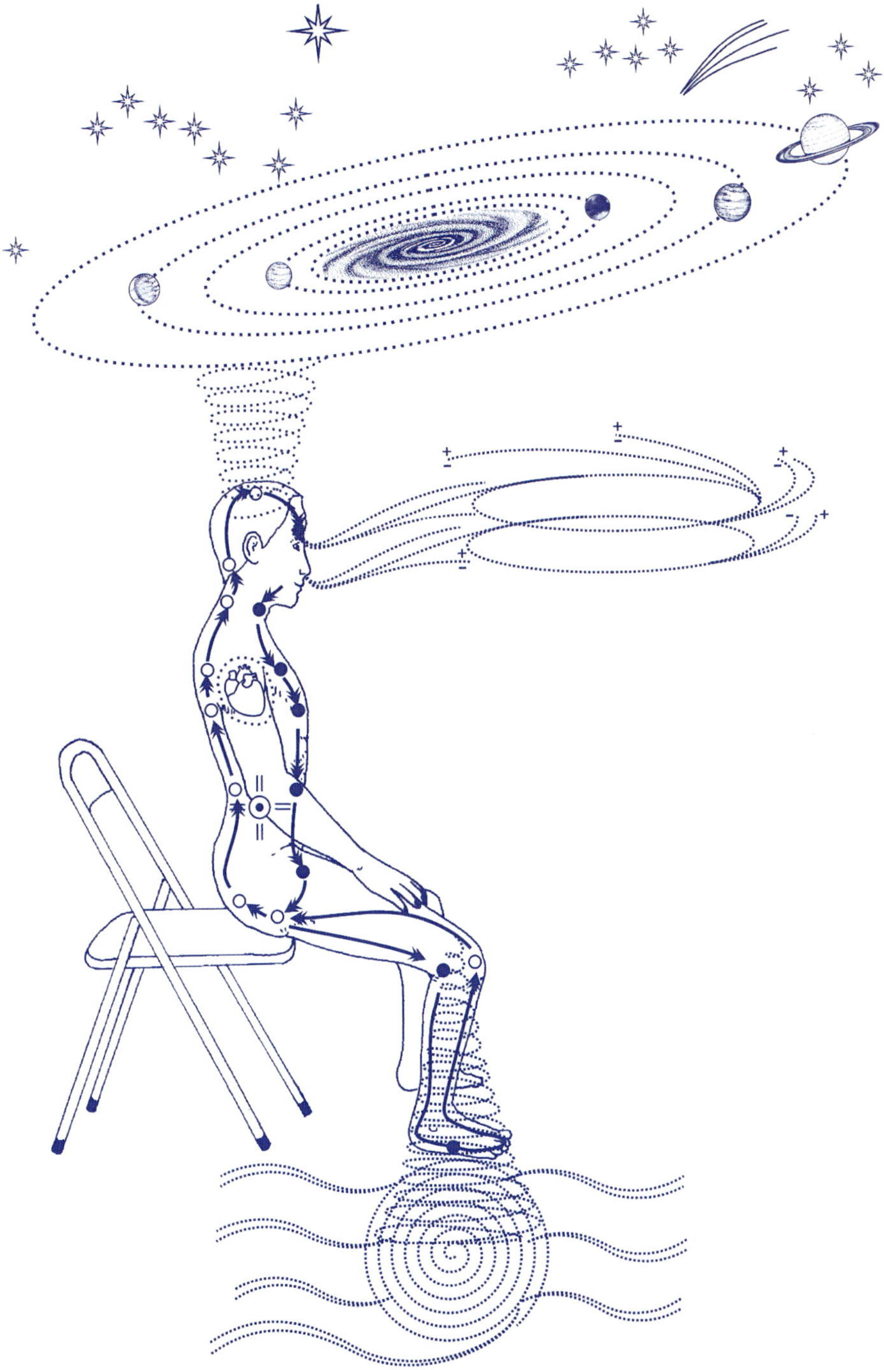

Fig. 8.8. The Microcosmic Orbit.

2. Focus on the chi in your navel center. Spiral the energy there. Then let it flow down to your sexual center (for women the Ovarian Palace, and for men the Sperm Palace, both of which are located at your pubic bone).
3. Now move the chi from your sexual center to your perineum (between your sexual organs and your anus) and then down to the soles of your feet.
4. Draw the chi up from the soles of your feet back to your perineum and then to your sacrum (the triangular bone that is connected to your tailbone).
5. Draw the chi from your sacrum up to the Door of Life, which is the point on the spine opposite the navel. You may need to take a sip of air to help you move the energy up each point up your back, neck, and head.
6. Draw the chi up to your midspine point (the T11 thoracic vertebra near the ribs).
7. Draw the energy up to the base of your skull (known as the Jade Pillow).
8. Draw the chi up to your crown, the middle of the top of your head.
9. Now move the energy from your crown back down to your mid-eyebrow point.
10. Lightly touch the tip of your tongue to the roof of your mouth. Press and release that point a few times. Then touch your upper palate again with your tongue and feel the electric or tingling feeling of chi in the tip of your tongue. Move the chi down from your mid-eyebrow point to the point where the tip of your tongue touches your palate.
11. Move the chi down from your palate to the center of your throat.
12. Move the energy from your throat to your heart center.
13. Move the chi from your heart center to your solar plexus (just below the bottom of your ribs) and feel a small sun shining out from that area.

14. Bring the energy back down to your navel.
15. Now circulate the energy through the entire sequence of points (steps 1 through 14) for a total of nine circulations. Breathe in as you move the chi up your back and breathe out as the energy flows down the front of your body.
16. Once the pathways are open, you can let your energy flow continuously like a river of energy without needing to stop at each point as you repeat the cycle. If you have an urge to use something addictive, think about that urge as you circulate the chi through the Microcosmic Orbit. Notice that the urge will lessen the more you circulate the energy (figure 8.8).

MANAGING SEXUAL ENERGY

Dopamine is a neurotransmitter, a chemical messenger that works in the brain. It facilitates the transmission of messages between nerve cells. Certain substances and activities will cause dopamine to flow much more powerfully than is natural. Examples include cocaine, gambling, carbohydrates, overuse of the internet, gaming, and sexual overindulgence. When someone is addicted to a substance or activity that stimulates a flood of dopamine into their system, they do not lose the desire for that same amount of dopamine even after they stop using whatever it is they're addicted to. If they're determined to stay clean and sober, the urge will try hard to reassert itself and find a new way to be satisfied.

Sexual activity is a common direction in which the need for dopamine is rerouted. To make matters more complicated, many people who have addictions have also absorbed the idea that their sexual urges are bad, sinful, shameful, or dirty, and they have either tried to suppress them or they just feel guilty when they have sexual urges. This results in even more pent-up sexual energy to manage.

The other common occurrence for people in recovery is that their sex drive will diminish or disappear altogether. People often feel depressed after they stop using whatever they're addicted to. Their bodies and minds seem to need to shut down a bit to recover from the abuse they suffered during active addiction. Some people, knowingly or not, have used sex to compensate for chronic depression. Having a low sex drive is a symptom of depression. A healthy and strong sex drive may not return without regulating the systems that feed it.

The Universal Healing Tao teaches people how to manage their sexual urges in healthy ways. Sexual energy is regarded in Taoism as a neutral energy—it's how it's used that determines whether it is positive or negative. Taoists consider sex to basically be something sacred, not shameful. The Universal Healing Tao recognizes that sexual energy is a powerful energy in the body, and so it focuses on harnessing that energy for the benefit of the whole body. We know that the sexual organs can produce powerful energy that can amplify what people feel. Therefore it's important to know how to regulate it and focus it properly. Otherwise, instead of warming the house it will burn it down, so to speak.

Rubbing on your sacrum with your hands is a simple way to start evening the flow of chi from your sexual organs. People who feel tension, pain, or a lack of circulation in the front part of their legs will often struggle with finding a solution. They can massage those areas, but that does not always solve the problem. When those areas are constricted, the energy flow between the sexual organs and the rest of the body is limited. The sacrum is the triangular-shaped bone at the base of your spine. In the Universal Healing Tao it is considered to be a sacred bone. It provides an energetic connection to the earth and is the beginning of our path to enlightenment, which ascends from the spine up to the crown. It has four holes on each side. Nerves thread through the holes and run from the back to the front. They end up in the pelvic floor. Rubbing your sacrum can stimulate the flow of energy from the back to the front. Put your fingertips on your sacrum and rub gently up and down for a minute or two. Notice that your

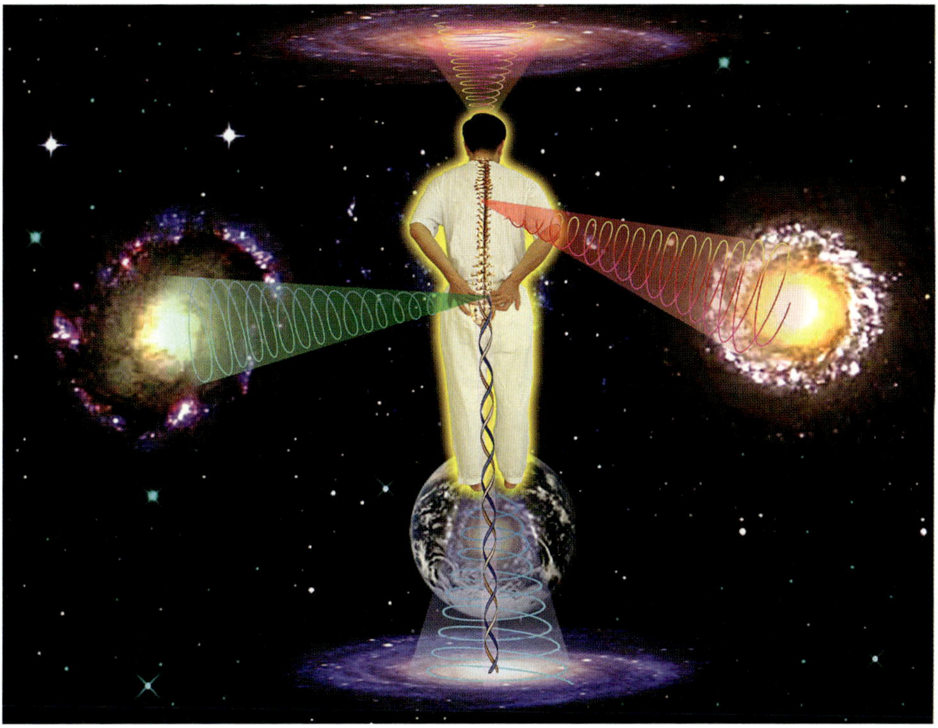

Fig. 8.9. Rub your sacrum to stimulate chi flow to your pelvic floor.

fingertips tingle after you stop. That's because you were making direct contact with the nerves in that area (figure 8.9).

A Taoist practice known as the Big Draw prevents sexual energy from getting too congested in the genitals and allows us to share that powerful energy with the rest of the body in ways that nourish and heal.

The Big Draw

The Big Draw practice is slightly different for men and women. The process for women will be described first. For both men and women it is best to do this practice during the daytime, as it is very stimulating and might make it difficult to sleep if you practice it at night.

First, the Big Draw for women (figure 8.10):

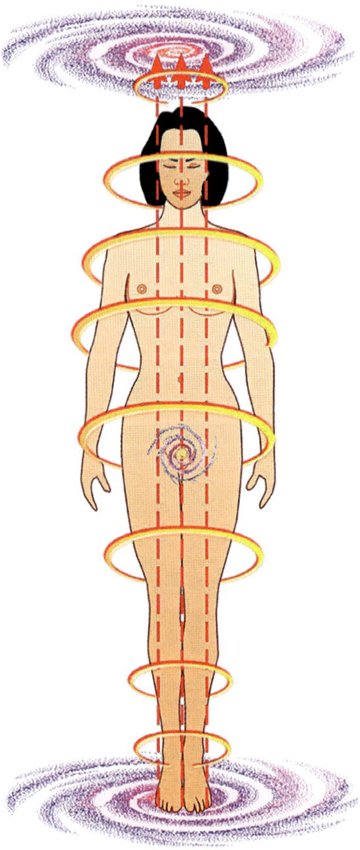

Fig. 8.10. The Big Draw practice for women can strengthen and heal the whole body. The practice can be performed while standing or sitting.

1. Focus on your vagina and clitoris. Picture them. If you don't know what they look like, get a mirror and look at them.
2. Lightly touch the lips of your vagina and clitoris until they start to get aroused.
3. Inhale gently but fully. Then when you exhale, lightly contract your vagina and squeeze around your clitoris.
4. Inhale again and release the squeeze around your clitoris. Picture your vagina expanding like a blossoming flower.
5. Repeat the process of exhaling and contracting, and then inhaling and releasing, nine to thirty-six times.
6. Now picture your uterus and ovaries also opening and closing like blossoming flowers.

7. Once you feel your sexual energy expanding, relax and draw the energy up your tailbone and sacrum and then up your spine to your brain. Make sure the chi passes through T11 (the thoracic spinal vertebra located near the ribs), C7 (the large cervical vertebra at the base of your neck), and the Jade Pillow point (located at the base of your skull) and ends up at your crown. If you have difficulty bringing the energy up, try contracting your vagina and your anus as you direct the orgasmic feeling up your spine to your brain.
8. Now allow the orgasmic energy to flow down throughout the rest of your body. You can also direct it to any part of your body that needs healing or strengthening.

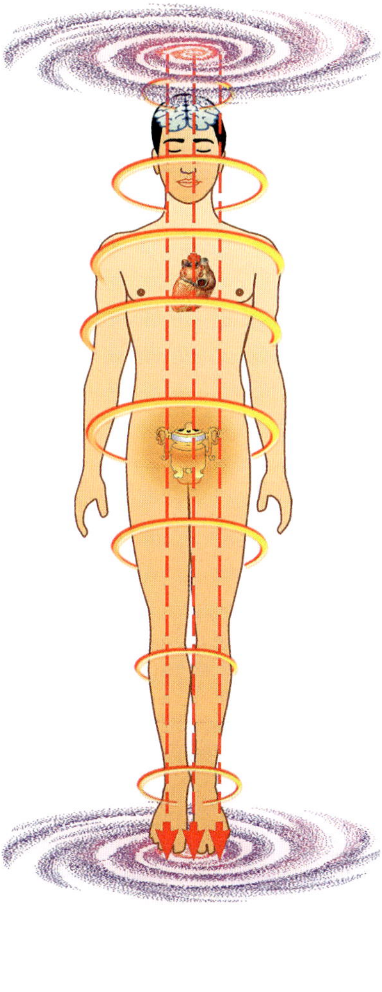

Fig. 8.11. The Big Draw practice for men nourishes the brain and then the whole body with creative chi from the sexual organs.

Now the Big Draw for men (figure 8.11):

1. Stand and touch your genitals until you have a strong erection. Stop at least thirty seconds before you reach the point where you would normally ejaculate.
2. Rest for a moment to regain control so you do not go past the point of no return and ejaculate. Now clamp your toes down on the floor and contract your pelvic floor muscle at the same time.
3. Squeeze your buttocks tightly and draw your sexual energy back from your perineum (between your sexual organs and your anus) toward your anus and spine.
4. Take a short inhalation and contract the muscles in your anus in waves to move the energy up your spine. This is similar to pumping the brakes on a car. You can rock your spine back and forth to help the energy travel up your spine.
5. Once the energy reaches the base of your skull (the Jade Pillow point), tuck your chin in gently and move the energy from your spine into your head.
6. Now roll your eyes up as if you are looking up into the top of your head. This will help to move the chi the rest of the way up to your crown.
7. Once you have pumped the chi up to your crown, you have completed one cycle of the Big Draw. You can measure how well you completed the practice by the state of your erection: as you draw the energy out of your genitals and up your spine your erection should decrease.
8. Repeat steps 3 through 6 eight more times.
9. Once you have pumped the energy up to the brain for a total of nine times, use your mind, your eyes, and your other senses to spiral the energy in your brain eighteen or thirty-six times. Spiral in both directions. Rest after doing that. Notice the feeling in your brain. Men often comment that they feel warmth and tingling in the brain when doing this practice.

10. When you feel that your brain is filled with that creative chi, touch the tip of your tongue to your palate and let the energy flow down the front channel that runs from your brain to the space between your eyebrows, then to your nose, throat, heart, and solar plexus, and lastly to your navel, where it can be stored.
11. Smile, and breathe slowly and gently in your lower abdomen. Focus on the vortex of energy there. Stay like that for at least one minute. After you have finished, try to maintain the same slow, gentle, and peaceful spirit as you continue with your day.

For those who have a reduced libido since going into recovery, the Universal Healing Tao has practices for that as well. First of all, massage can stimulate the energy from the sexual organs. Men should massage their testicles. Massaging them enhances male potency and activates the production of healthy sperm. It's also a simple way to energize yourself when you are tired during the day. Both men and women can massage their breasts. The practice begins with touching the nipples and slowly making spiral motions around them, starting from the nipple and working to the outside. Feel the connection between your nipples and your sexual organs. Then continue making spiraling motions with your fingers as you move your hands slowly down the nipple line toward your groin area. Make nine spirals with your fingers on the way down to your groin Find your sensitive spots and spiral over them. Feel the energy moving, warming, tingling, and spreading in each area. Feeling the energy is very important. Sometimes when you feel the energy, the energy rises up to the brain all by itself.

Scrotal and vaginal compression can also help men and women enhance their libido. Try the following:

Scrotal and Vaginal Compression

1. To prepare, first do the Crane Neck practice and Spinal Cord Rocking. Spinal Cord Rocking involves sitting on a chair and then

rocking slowly from side to side so that the tissues that are connected to the bones that make contact with the seat of the chair are massaged (see chapter 5 for Spinal Cord Rocking and chapter 6 for the Crane Neck practice).

2. Rub your chest to make sure that region does not feel constricted. Now inhale, contract your sexual organs and anus, and use your toes like claws to grasp the ground tightly. Take a deep breath and hold it. Press against your lower abdomen just above the pubic bone with your fingers.
3. Exhale and breathe the energy down to either your uterus or your testicles.
4. Hold your breath. Now pull your perineum up very strongly and press down more with your fingers.
5. Inhale and rock your body to the left and right. Release your fingers. Feel your testicles or uterus "breathing." It feels like they are expanding and contracting with each breath that you take.
6. Repeat steps 2–5, but this time press against the upper part of your Lower Tan Tien with your fingers when you press the energy down. Do this a few times. Rock your body again from left to right.
7. Rest. Smile at your sexual organs and let the energy rise up to your brain and then back to your navel. Feel your sexual organs breathing together with your brain. Notice how charged with energy they feel.

CONSERVING SEXUAL ENERGY AS WE AGE

Conserving sexual energy becomes more important as we age, when the ability to produce sexual energy decreases as the body's systems slow down. If you use up too much sexual energy, the body will become very tired and will age prematurely. Men lose sexual energy through ejaculation. Women mostly lose sexual energy through menstruation and childbearing. The sexual organs can create a lot of energy, but they cannot store it efficiently. It must be discharged if it is not stored. Learning how to conserve sexual energy is important in recovery not only so that people can feel vibrant and energetic, but also so they can have enough energy to get through all of the work it takes to transform their lives in ways that support recovery and healthy living. To accomplish this, men need to learn the difference between orgasm and ejaculation. Ejaculation occurs when sperm is released from the head of the penis. Orgasm is the energetic explosion that happens inside a man prior to ejaculation. If a man can learn how to have an orgasm without having to ejaculate, then he does not lose that powerful energy. It can be maintained, cultivated over repeated orgasms and circulated through the Microcosmic Orbit to benefit the whole body.

Conserving Male Sexual Energy

1. Start by lubricating your penis.
2. Before focusing on your genitals, remember to touch and massage the rest of your body, especially your stomach, thighs, and nipples.
3. Self-pleasure in whatever way works for you. Remember to stimulate your entire penis, your scrotum, and your perineum.
4. Pay close attention to your arousal rate. Notice your increasing levels of arousal. Be aware of any tingling at the root of your penis, the stages of erection, changes in your breathing, and the speed of your heartbeat.
5. As you feel yourself getting close the point of no return, stop pleasuring yourself and lightly contract your PC muscle around your prostate. You can also delay ejaculation by pressing on the tip of your penis or by using your mind to squeeze it. The important thing is to learn how to pay close attention to your rate of arousal and stop in time so that you do not ejaculate, at least a few strokes before the point of no return.
6. If you feel that your sexual energy is becoming too hard to control, draw that energy up your spine with your mind and squeeze

and release your PC muscle several times. If that does not get your arousal level under control, then stop for ten or twenty seconds and focus on deep breathing.

7. Notice the contraction that occurs in your PC muscle and anus that happens at the contractile phase of orgasm, which is just before orgasm.
8. Stop after your sexual energy has peaked several times without ejaculating. You will feel peaceful and energized. Notice how your sexual energy feels as it circulates through your body. It may feel tingly, itchy, or prickly.

Conserving Female Sexual Energy

For women, a drilled jade egg* is used in this practice. A string of unwaxed dental floss is threaded through the hole that passes through the egg. Do not use waxed dental floss to thread through it, as the practice creates warmth in the vagina and could melt the wax coating. The string helps with the removal of the egg. The preferred material for the egg is jade because it is sturdy, smooth, and nonporous. Wooden eggs or any eggs that have a painted or chemical finish should definitely be avoided (figure 8.12).

In the beginning, practice with the egg should be done in the morning as this practice can be very stimulating, and practicing at night might lead to sleeplessness. Make sure the egg is clean; it should be boiled prior to first using and washed every time after that and placed in its own bag or container.

1. Begin with the breast massage described earlier: touch your nipples and slowly make spiral motions around your breasts. Feel the connection between your nipples and your sexual organs. Then continue making spiraling motions with your fingers as you move your hands

*You can purchase a drilled jade egg from MantakChia.com. They are available in different sizes, and jade comes in different colors.

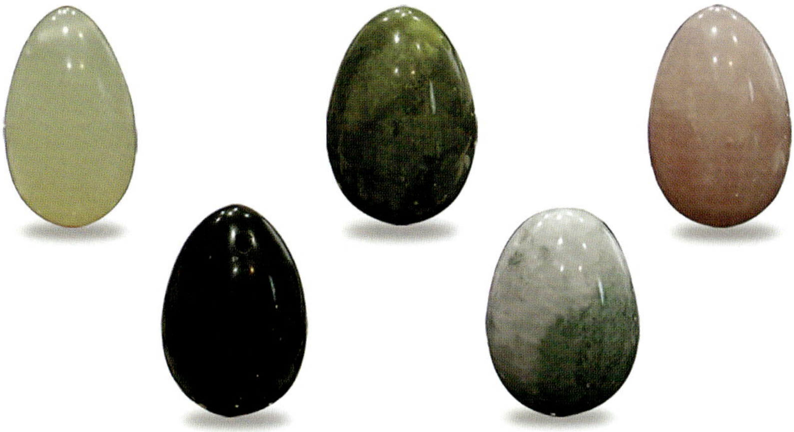

Fig. 8.12. Jade eggs come in different colors. The Jade Egg practice can help women balance their hormones, strengthen their pelvic floor, and build strong sexual energy. The practice can be performed while standing or sitting, but most women find it easier to start while lying down.

slowly down the nipple line toward your groin area. Make nine spirals with your fingers on the way down to your groin. As you make those nine spirals, find your sensitive spots and spiral over them. Feel the energy moving, warming, tingling, and spreading in each area.

2. Rub your hands together and place each hand over its respective ovary. Your ovaries are the breadth of one hand below the navel on each side of your abdomen. Massage your ovaries thirty-six times in both directions. Once you are sufficiently stimulated, the warm, moist vaginal secretions indicate that your body is ready for the egg to be inserted. If you cannot reach that level of lubrication on your own, lubricate the egg with a nontoxic oil or gel prior to inserting. Be sure that the lubricant is not petroleum-based.
3. Insert the egg into your vagina, wide side first with the string closest to the entrance to your vagina. After some practice you should be able to increase the suction force sufficiently to pull it in with your vaginal muscles. Once it is inside, stand with your feet parallel and

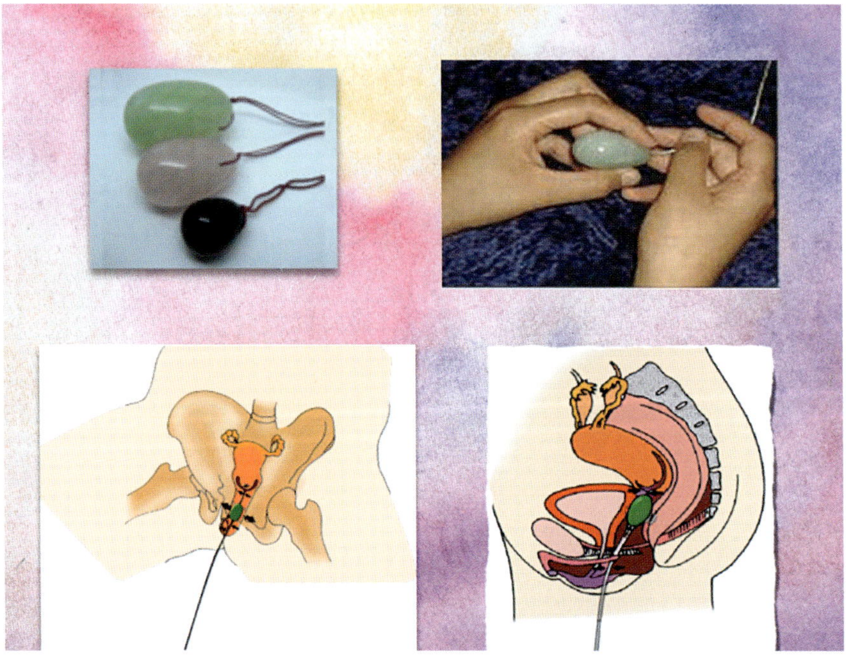

Fig 8.13. Moving the egg up and down, the yoni egg practice.

shoulder-width apart. Keep your knees slightly bent. Lift your arms up in front of you to the level of your solar plexus. at a 45-degree angle. Your palms face upward. Clench your fists.

4. Focus on and contract the vaginal muscles to close the vaginal orifice.
5. Inhale slowly and deeply down into your ovaries as you gather your sexual energy there. Now draw that energy down through your uterus to your clitoris and hold it there.
6. Contract and hold your lower, middle, and upper vaginal muscles so that the egg is pushed into your vaginal canal. Ideally you will contract from your uterus and bladder. Move your eyes upward and focus your mind to make the movement of the energy as smooth as possible.
7. Move the egg back and forth through the three sections of the vagina by contracting and releasing your vaginal muscles in combi-

nation with gently tugging and releasing the string that is attached to the egg. As you do this, hold onto the string with a slight tension and use this counterpressure along with your vaginal muscles to help the process (figure 8.13).

8. Gradually squeeze the middle canal to establish a grip on the egg as you increase the pressure to move it up and down the canal at will.
9. Gradually increase the speed of the up and down motion. Then maintain that pace until you feel the need to rest. Resting afterward is important so that chi can accumulate. Now take a deep breath and draw the accumulated energy into the Microcosmic Orbit (described earlier in this chapter).
10. Remove the egg. You may need to contract your vaginal muscles to do this. At first a squatting position may be necessary. You can also elevate one leg on a chair to facilitate the removal. Simply pull it out using the attached string, but keep in mind that one of the purposes of the egg practice is also to build up the muscles inside to prevent urinary and energy leakage.
11. Massage your perineum, your mons (the mound of fatty tissue covering your pubic area), and your coccyx (tailbone). Massaging after using the egg is very important to make sure that the remaining energy is cleared so that your body can absorb it easily. Now gently tap your lower abdomen with your palm to remove excess energy from your ovaries, vagina, and clitoris.
12. Rest. Practice the Microcosmic Orbit meditation to circulate the energy you have generated throughout your body. You can also practice the Six Healing Sounds meditation found in chapter 9 to cool your body down.

FOOD AS MEDICINE

When someone is in active addiction they usually do not pay enough attention to making sure they have a good diet. If you don't know how to balance your diet to fit your individual needs, you can end up feeling restless, irritable, or just *off*. If that feeling lasts long enough it can trigger your urge to feed your addiction, because that's the only way your body knows how to make itself feel better.

It is also common for people to end up eating too much or eating too many carbohydrates when they are trying to stay sober. Trying to figure out what foods and food combinations are best can be very confusing. There are so many diets, programs, and fads that claim to have the answers. Taoists have been studying how to use food to balance the energies in the body for millennia. When we absorb chi from food it becomes our own chi.

Another important aspect of healthy eating involves the idea of acid-alkaline balance as defined by Western nutrition. Acid in this context means an acid-forming effect in the body, while alkaline refers to an alkalizing effect in the body. Though there are some differences between the two approaches, East and West, in general we can say that alkaline is yin, and acid is yang. We need both acid and alkaline, both yin and yang. Meats, sugars, pasta, grains, and processed foods are all classified as acidic, with some tap water and processed foods and meats being the most acidic of all. However, a great assortment of vegetables and fruits are alkaline.

Acid, or yang energy, can be compared to the gasoline that fuels a car, while alkaline, or yin energy, can be compared to the oil needed to lubricate the parts of the car and thin down some of the glutinous, sticky fluids. Indeed, yin energy is necessary for the blood, joints, and connective tissue, and for ensuring the smooth working of the body. Yin energy nourishes the body in order for it to save energy; it has a weight-losing effect and increases energy input. Yang energy, in contrast, increases energy output, so a physically active job means you need a greater quantity of yang than you would need in a sedentary job. Both yin and yang together dictate how what we eat affects our metabolism—or rather the balance of the two does. As people get older and the level of their physical activity decreases, they obviously need less yang food. This change in the level of activity signals a change in the metabolism.

Today the consumption of meat as well as fast foods, sweets, processed foods, preserved foods, canned foods, liquor, all of which are acid, is much greater than ever in the West, so in general our diet leans heavily toward the acid side. Anyone who has been involved in using addictive substances is in all likelihood extremely acidic. In overly acid conditions the body becomes more and more polluted, while digestion becomes less and less efficient. We cannot acquire enough energy from what we eat, resulting in fatigue and muscle aches and pains. The constant demand for energy that cannot be absorbed from food causes the metabolism to run amok and not work efficiently, further aggravating the urge to indulge in the addictive substance. In addition, high levels of acidity impede motor activity, which makes you tire easily when engaging in physical activity. Excessive acidity has other associated problems. Negative thoughts arise and nightmares can occur. Moreover, the liver has to work extra hard to filter out and remove the accumulated toxins, requiring large amounts of energy that are taken away from the rest of the body, contributing further to chronic exhaustion.

A good balance of food intake would be 20 to 30 percent acid food and 70 to 80 percent alkaline food. ". . . all watery type fruits, vegetables, and their juices are classified as alkaline quality foods. Acid quality foods are all proteins, starches, fats, and sugars; that is, all nuts, seeds, cheeses, bread, potatoes, rice, oils, and dried and sweet fruit, like dates, raisins, figs, and bananas. All heavy type foods are acid-forming." (*Cosmic Nutrition: The Taoist Approach to Health and Longevity*, by Mantak Chia and William U. Wei, 2012) A good place to start rebalancing your diet is to concentrate on making sure your meals have a mixture of the five colors of healthy foods to stimulate the energies in each of your yin organs. Red foods (like beets, for example) will nourish your heart. Yellow foods (like yellow beans or squash) are good for your spleen. Food that is white in color (like rice, for example) helps the energy in your lungs. Blue or dark-colored food (such as meat or dark-colored mushrooms) helps your kidneys. Green food (such as spinach, kale, or green beans) nourishes your liver.

For detailed information on how to eat according to the Universal Healing Tao, see Master Chia's book *Taoist Secrets of Eating for Balance: Your Personal Program for Five-Element Nutrition*.

9

Practices for a Full and Restful Sleep

Life during active addiction is stressful. Once someone enters recovery it is still stressful because now they have to reevaluate and rebalance their life without the crutch their addiction provided. Stress creates friction and heat in the body. Heat rises. It can only rise as far as the head, where it whirls around, making it difficult to calm down and stop obsessing over problems and get to sleep. Poor sleep lowers dopamine levels in the brain, which can then trigger the desire to return to the powerful source of dopamine found previously in the addictive substance or activity that the person is trying to avoid. This is when the temptation to return to one's addiction can come up. The Six Healing Sounds is a nighttime practice that cools and detoxifies the yin organs, which allows the body to slow down and the mind to settle in preparation for deep sleep.

The Six Healing Sounds

Lung Sound: First Healing Sound

The lung sound is a metal sound. It resembles the vibrating sound of a bell. It activates the lung chi.

Associated organ: large intestine

Element: metal

Season: autumn

Color: white

Emotions: grief, sadness, loss, depression

Virtues: courage, justice, righteousness

Senses: smell, touch

Taste: pungent

Related parts of the body: chest, inner arms, thumbs

Sound: *sssssssss*, with your teeth together and your tongue behind your teeth; pull the corners of your mouth back.

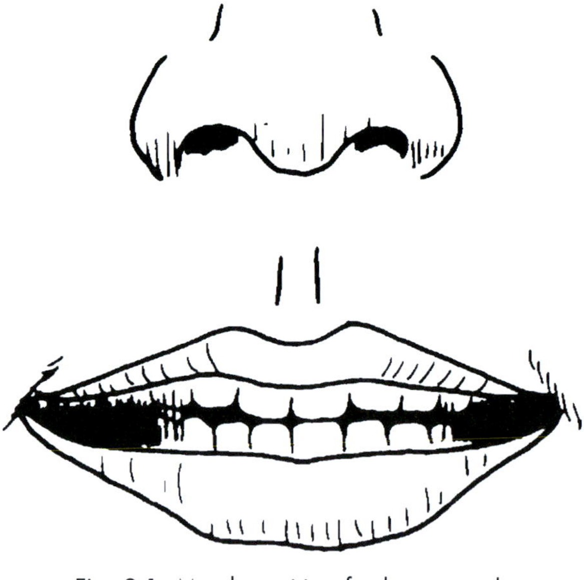

Fig. 9.1. Mouth position for lung sound.

1. Sit on the edge of a chair with your back straight, your palms resting on your lungs (figure 9.2).

   Close your eyes. Smile at your lungs. Notice the quality of energy in your lungs. See a white light around your lungs. See it fresh and pure, like the energy of the mountains. Hear the metal sound.
2. Take a deep breath in, open your eyes, and raise your arms out in front of you with your palms still facing your lungs. Raise your arms until your palms are at eye level. Then rotate your palms outward and bring them above your head until they face upward. The fingers on each hand should point to those on the other hand. Keep your elbows rounded and out to the sides. Do not straighten your arms. Close your jaws and gently clench your teeth. Close your lips softly and make the sound *sssssssss* through your teeth

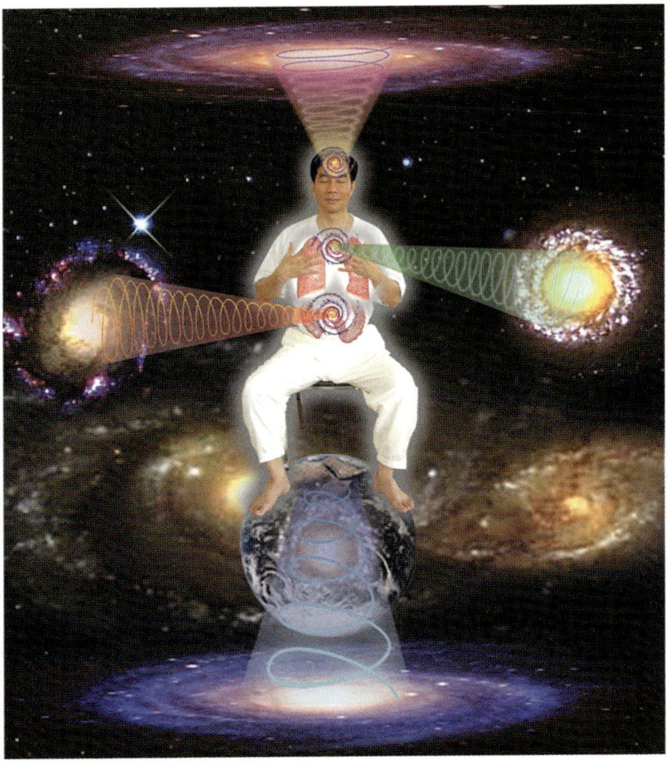

Fig. 9.2. Notice what you are feeling in and around your lungs.

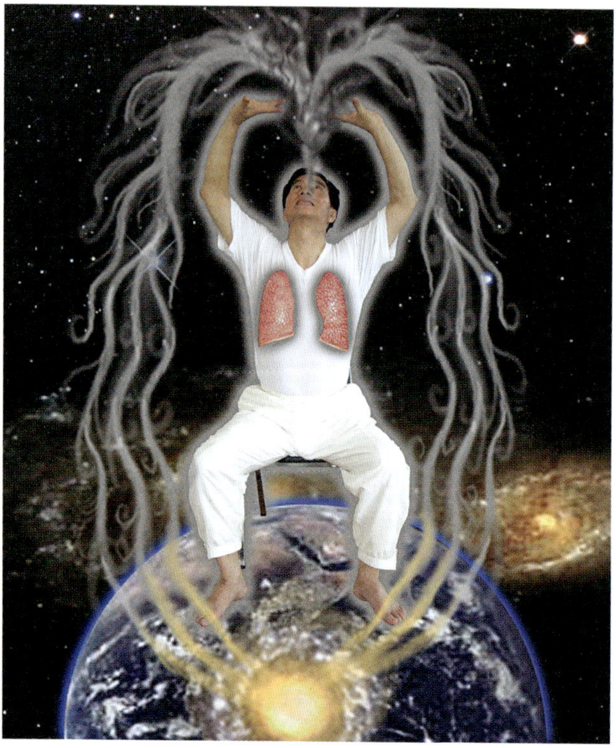

Fig. 9.3. Performing the lung sound.

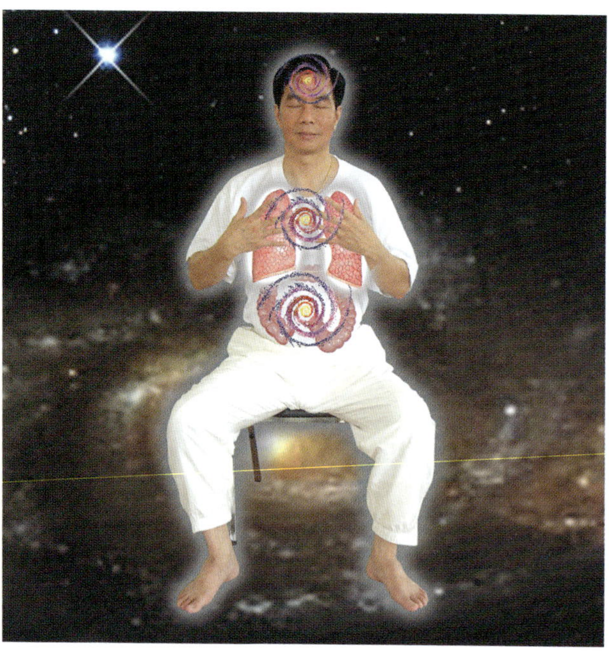

Fig. 9.4. Pour white light down from your crown to your lungs.

as you slowly and fully exhale. When you first start practicing this meditation you can make the sound out loud. Eventually you can make the sound subvocally, meaning that you are making the sound so quietly that only you can hear it. Feel the sound move the chi in your lungs. Know that as you make the lung sound, any excess heat and toxins are expelled from the lungs as the sacs that surround the lungs are compressed while you make the sound (figure 9.3).

3. Once you've exhaled completely, turn your palms over and scoop up the white light from around your head and pour that light from your crown down into your lungs. Now lower your arms and hold your hands in front of your lungs. Radiate the white light into your lungs (figure 9.4).
4. Close your eyes and rest. Focus on your lungs. Smile into them and imagine that you are still making the lung sound. Feel the vibration of the sound moving and cleaning the energy in your lungs. Breathe normally and see your lungs glowing with a bright white light. Now they have been strengthened, and the qualities of courage and righteousness have been activated in them. As you continue to breathe, try to feel that fresh, white metal energy is replacing excess hot, toxic, depressed energy (figure 9.5 on page 186).
5. Take some time to get in touch with your lungs and to nurture good emotions in them. This is the most important part of this practice. Once you have expelled and released hot, toxic energy from them, there is room for good emotional qualities to grow. Concentrate on the feelings of courage and righteousness as you transform any grief, sadness, loss, and depression in your lungs. Sit up straight and tall so you can feel courageous and try to maintain the feeling of the lung sound for increasingly longer periods after each practice and in your daily life.
6. Repeat this sequence three to six times. For sadness, colds, flu, toothaches, asthma, emphysema, or depression consider repeating this exercise six, nine, twelve, or twenty-four times.

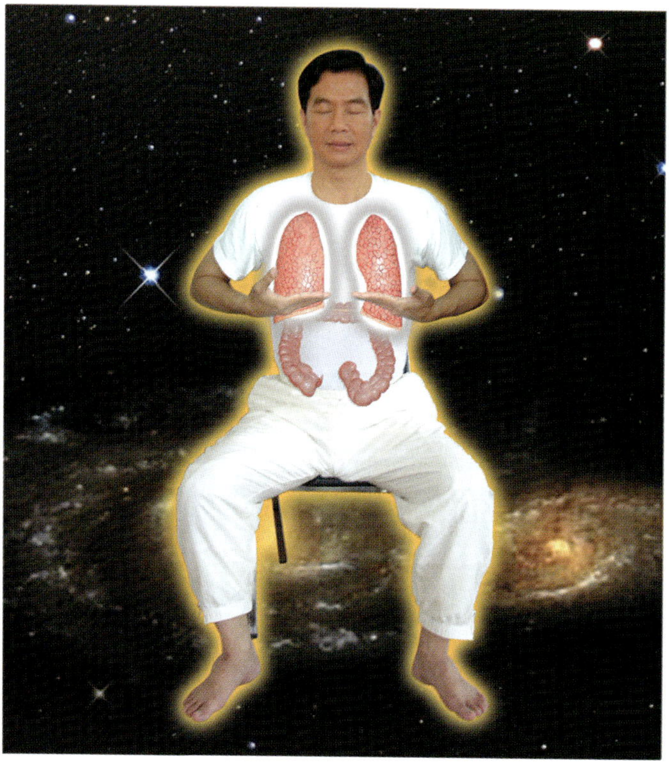

Fig. 9.5. Smile at your lungs.

Kidney Sound: Second Healing Sound

The kidney sound is a water sound that activates the kidney chi.

Associated organ: bladder
Element: water
Season: winter
Color: dark blue
Emotions: fear, stress, anxiety
Virtues: gentleness, calmness, alertness, stillness
Sense: hearing
Taste: salty
Related parts of the body: sides of the feet, inner legs, chest
Sound: *chooooooo* with your lips forming an *O*, like when you blow out a candle (figure 9.6)

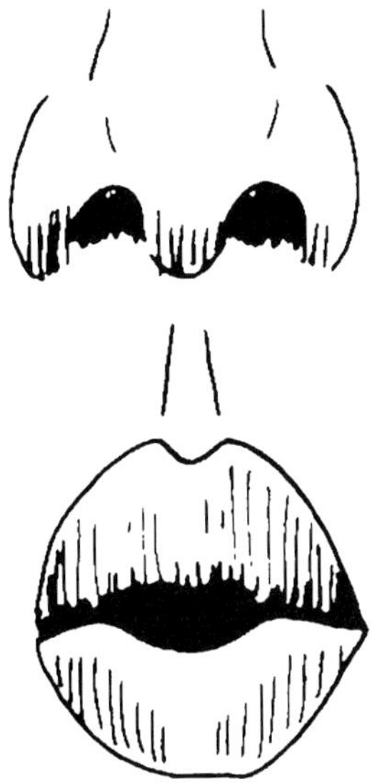

Fig. 9.6. Round your lips to make the sound that people make when they blow out a candle.

1. Sit on the edge of a chair with your back straight, resting your hands on your kidneys. Close your eyes. Smile down at your kidneys. Notice the quality of energy in your kidneys. See a blue light around them. Think about the sun shining on the water of your kidneys, warming and healing their energy (figure 9.7).
2. Take a deep breath. Now open your eyes and bring your legs together with your knees and ankles touching. Lean forward and clasp the fingers of both hands together around your knees. Bend your torso forward until your arms are straight. Allow your back to round and protrude in the area of your kidneys. Keep your arms straight and tilt your head up until you can look straight ahead. Feel the pull on your spine.
3. Round your lips and slightly exhale as you make the kidney sound, *choooooooo*. While making the sound, contract your abdomen by pulling it in toward your kidneys. At first you can make the kidney sound out loud, but eventually you will be able to make it subvocally. Feel the chi in your kidneys start to move when you make the sound. Any excess heat and toxins are

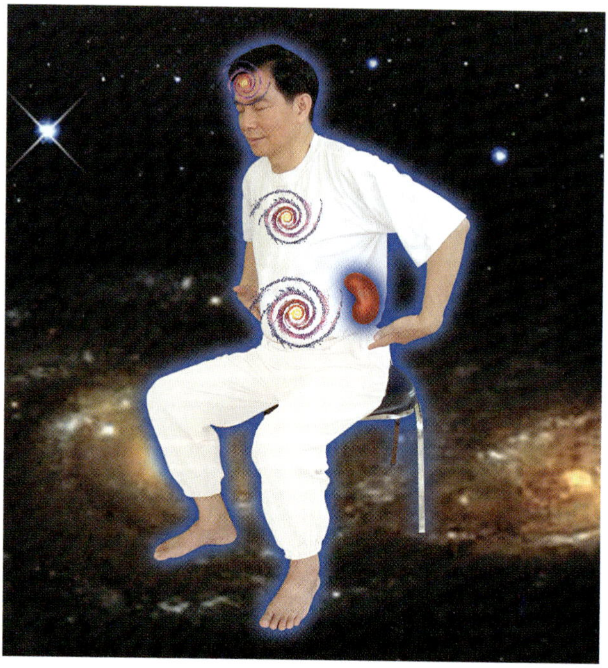

Fig. 9.7. Smile at your kidneys.

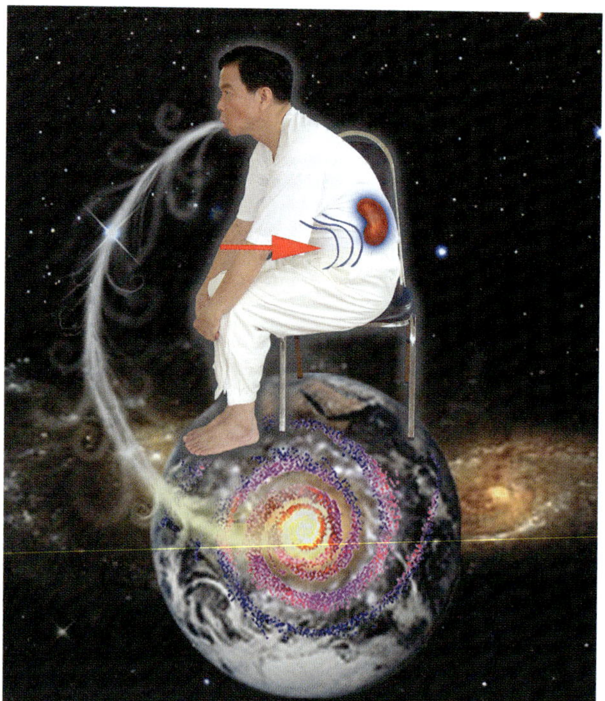

Fig. 9.8. Make the kidney sound, *chooooooo*.

expelled from the kidneys as the sacs surrounding the kidneys are compressed (figure 9.8).

4. After you have fully exhaled, sit up straight, separate your legs, move your arms up to the height of your crown, and scoop up blue light. Pour that light down over your body and into your kidneys with a sweeping gesture of the hands. Allow that blue light to radiate in your kidneys, which will enhance the kidney virtues of gentleness, calmness, and stillness.
5. Place your palms on your kidneys. Rest. Close your eyes and focus on your kidneys. Smile at them and imagine that you are still making the kidney sound. Feel the vibration of the sound as it moves and cleans the energy in your kidneys.
6. Breathe normally and see your kidneys glowing with a cool blue light. This strengthens your kidneys and the virtues in them. With each breath, try to feel that bright blue water energy is replacing hot, toxic, fearful energy.
7. Nurture good emotions. This is the most important part of the practice. Take all the time you need to get in touch with your kidneys. As you cool off excess heat and let cool water energy expand in your kidneys, good emotional qualities will have room to grow there. Concentrate on the feelings of gentleness, calmness, stillness, and alertness as you transform fear in your kidneys. Notice that your lower back relaxes and your willpower increases when you do this exercise. Try to maintain the feelings and sensations of the transformed energy for increasingly longer periods after each practice and in your daily life (figure 9.9 on page 190).
8. Repeat the sequence three to six times or more to alleviate fear, fatigue, dizziness, ringing in the ears, or back pain.

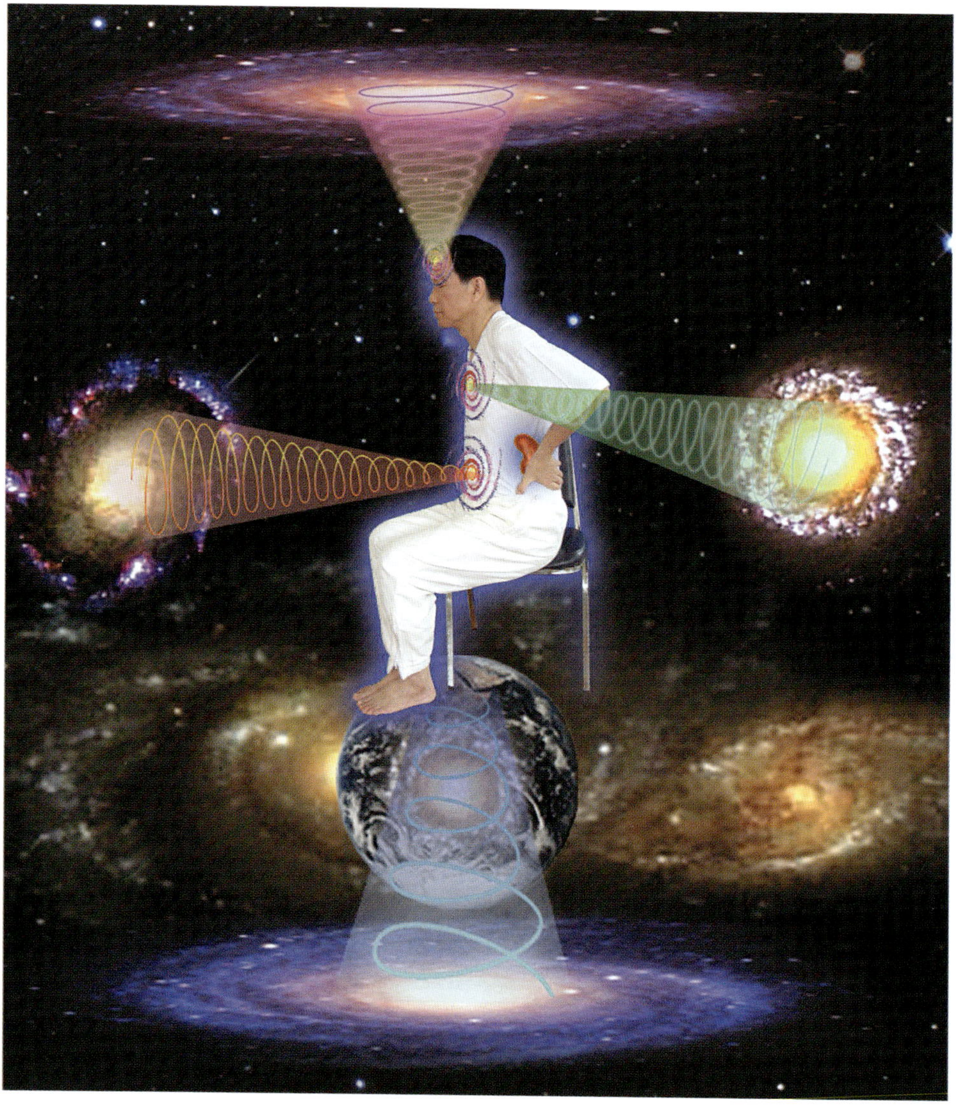

Fig. 9.9. Gather energy into your kidneys.

Liver Sound: Third Healing Sound

The liver sound is a wood sound. It activates the liver's chi.

Associated organ: gallbladder
Element: wood
Season: spring
Color: green
Emotions: anger, frustration, jealousy, envy, resentment
Virtues: generosity, forgiveness, kindness
Sense: sight
Taste: bitter
Related parts of the body: inner legs, groin, diaphragm, ribs
Sound: *shhhhhhh* with your tongue near your upper palate

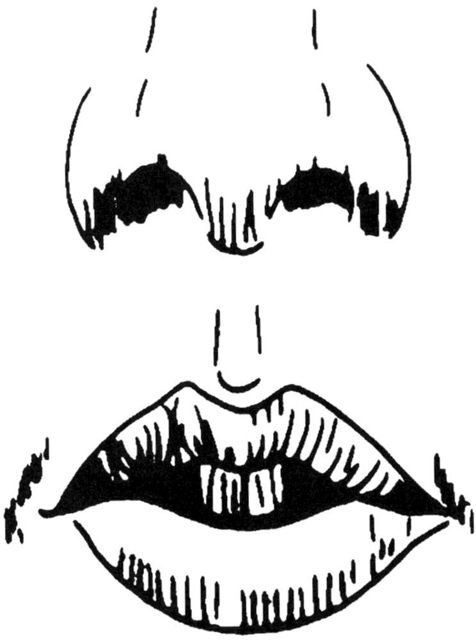

Fig. 9.10. To make the liver sound, exhale with your tongue near your upper palate.

1. Sit comfortably with your back straight. Place your palms on your liver. Close your eyes. Smile down at your liver and connect with it. Notice the quality of the energy in your liver. Picture a big green forest in your liver. See the sun shining on the forest, creating life force and bright green light (figure 9.11).
2. Take a deep breath, open your eyes, and extend your arms out to your sides with palms facing up. Slowly raise your arms to the level of your crown. Follow the movements of your arms with your eyes. Interlace your fingers and rotate your joined hands until they face the ceiling, palms up. Push up with heels of your hands. Stretch your arms out. Your elbows should be pushing toward the back.
3. Bend slightly to the left, which exerts a gentle pull on your liver. Open your eyes wider. They are energetically connected to your liver. Slowly exhale and make the liver sound: *shhhhhhhh*.

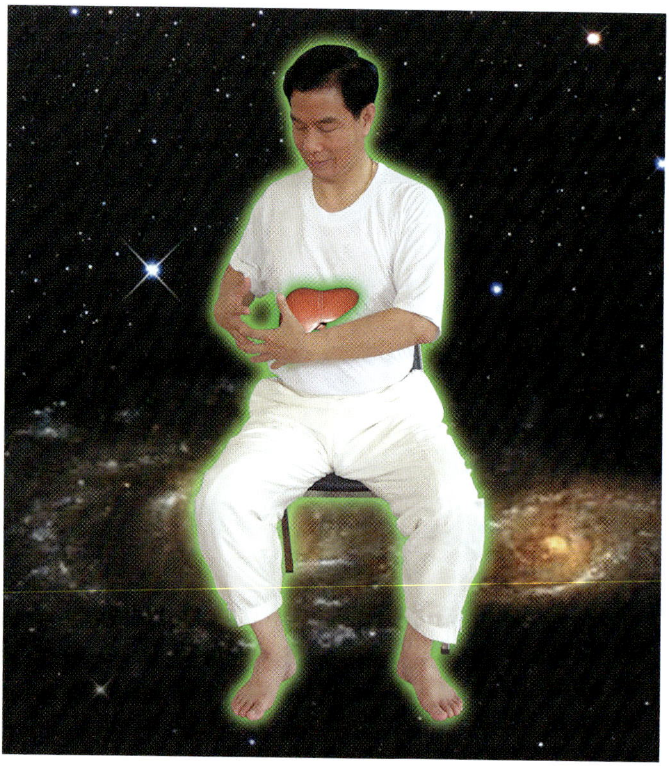

Fig. 9.11. Smile at your liver.

You can make the sound out loud at first. Eventually you will be able to make it subvocally. Feel the sound start to move the energy in the liver, and feel the excess heat and toxins being expelled from the liver as the sac around it is compressed (figure 9.12).

4. After you have fully exhaled, sit up straight, separate your hands, and scoop up green light into your palms. Pour that light over your body and into your liver. Allow green forest energy and kindness to radiate into your liver.
5. Slowly bring your palms back to your liver. Rest. Smile. Close your eyes and focus on your liver. Imagine that you are still making the liver sound. Feel the vibration of the sound moving and cleaning the energy in your liver.
6. Breathe normally. See your liver glowing with rejuvenating green light. This strengthens your liver and activates the virtues in it.

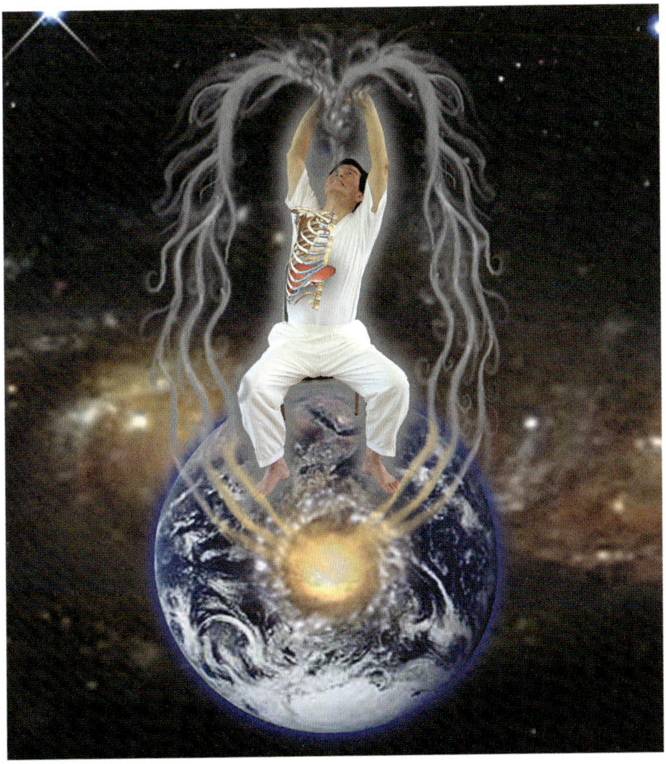

Fig. 9.12. Make the liver sound.

With each breath, try to feel the bright green wood energy replacing excess hot, toxic, angry, frustrated, and aggressive energy in your liver (figure 9.13).

7. Nurture good emotions. This is the most important part of this practice. Take all the time you need to connect with your liver. As you remove the excess heat and allow warm, moist, green wood energy to expand in your liver, kindness and generosity will have room to grow. Concentrate on the virtues of kindness and forgiveness as you transform anger and aggression in your liver. Feel warm and energized, and maintain those feelings for as long as you can after you complete the exercise (figure 9.14).
8. Repeat the sequence three to six times. Practice more to expel anger, to clear red or watery eyes, to remove a sour or bitter taste in your mouth, and to detoxify your liver.

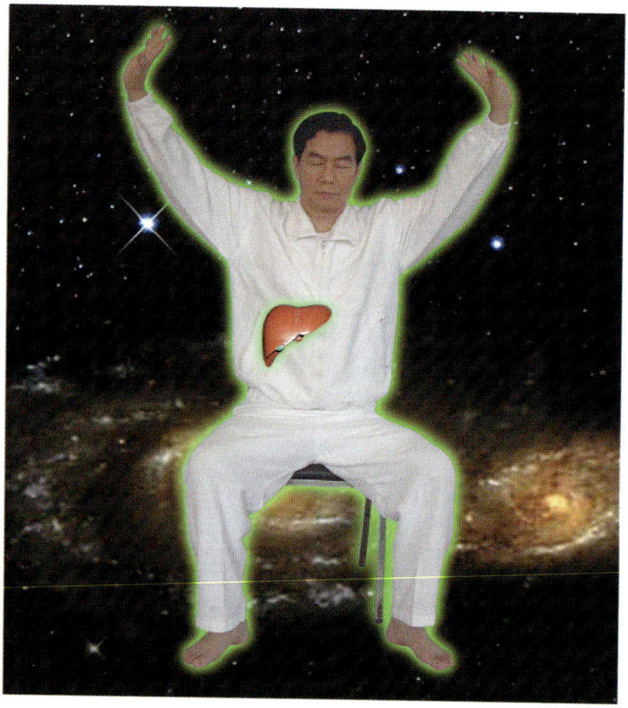

Fig. 9.13. Scoop green forest light and pour it into your liver.

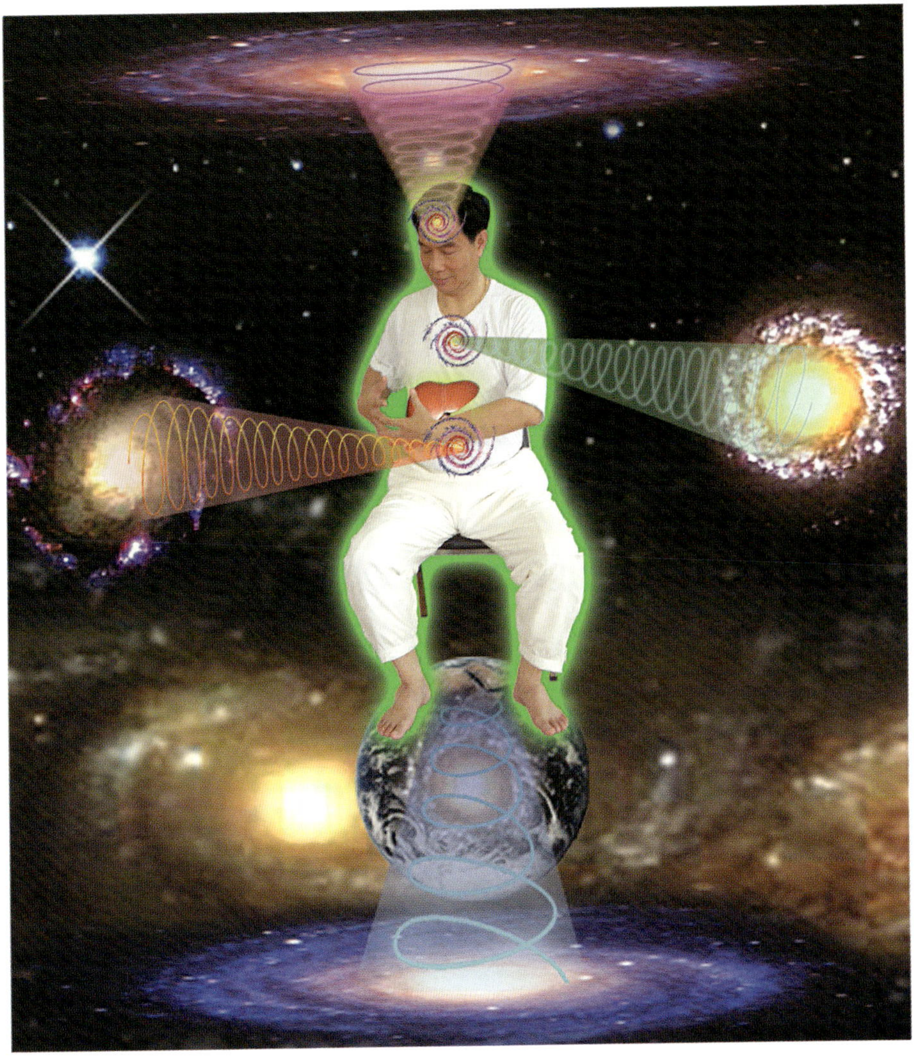

Fig. 9.14. Gather bright green wood energy into your liver.

Heart Sound: Fourth Healing Sound

The heart sound is a fire sound that activates the heart's energy.

Associated organ: small intestine

Element: fire

Season: summer

Color: red

Emotions: hastiness, arrogance, cruelty

Virtues: joy, honor, sincerity, love

Related parts of the body: armpits, inner arms

Senses: taste

Taste: bitter

Sound: *hawwwwww*, with your mouth wide open

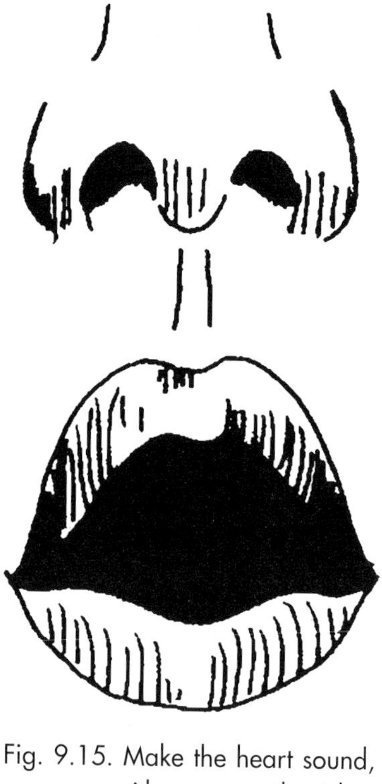

Fig. 9.15. Make the heart sound, *hawwwwww*, with your mouth wide open.

1. Sit comfortably on the edge of a chair with your back straight. Rest your hands in front of your heart. Close your eyes. Smile down to your heart and make a connection with it. Notice the quality of the energy in your heart. Think about a sunset on the ocean that produces a reddish light (figure 9.16).
2. Take a deep breath, open your eyes, and interlace your fingers and raise your arms overhead like you did for the liver sound. However, unlike the liver sound, this time you will lean slightly to the right to gently stretch your heart area located just slightly to the left of the center of your chest.

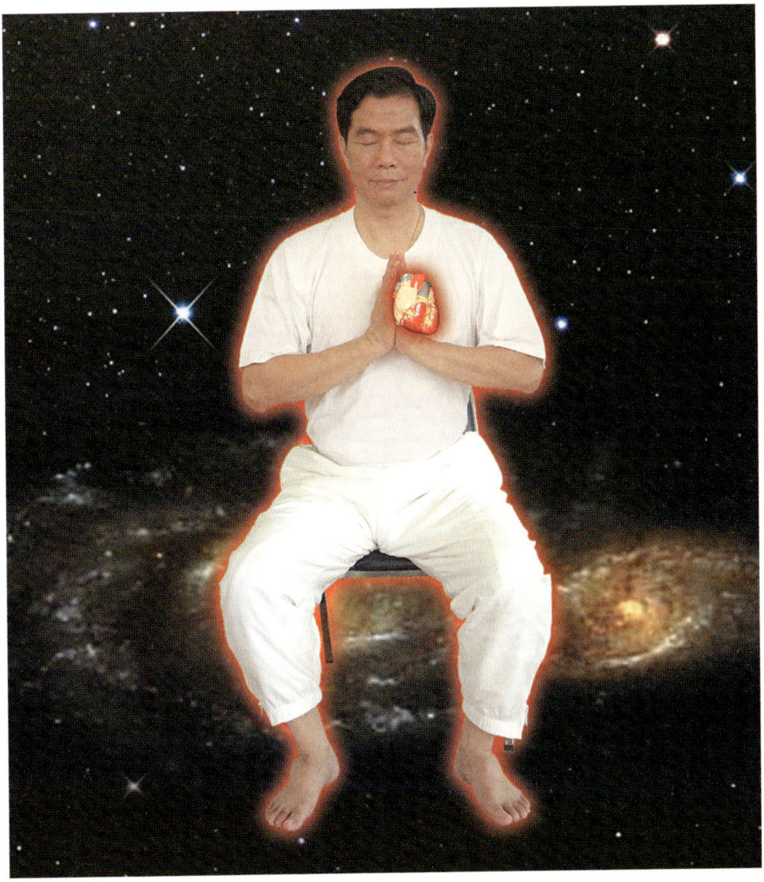

Fig. 9.16. Smile into your heart.

3. Focus on your heart. Feel the connection between your tongue to your open mouth. Inhale, round your lips, and make the sound *hawwwwww* while you slowly exhale. The first few times you practice this sound you may need to make the sound out loud. Over time you will gain the ability to make it subvocally. Feel the sound start to move the energy in your heart. Feel the excess heat and toxins being expelled from your heart as the pericardium sac around it is compressed when you make the sound (figure 9.17).
4. After you have fully exhaled, sit erect, separate your hands, and scoop red light into your palms. Pour that light over your body and into your heart. Slowly bring your arms down, palms facing out. Scoop up more red light and then hold both of your hands in front of your heart. Let the red light, love, and inner joy radiate into your heart (figure 9.18).
5. Bring your hands back in front of your heart. Rest. Close your eyes. Focus on your heart. Smile at your heart and imagine that you are still making the heart sound. Feel the energy of the sound moving and cleaning the energy in your heart. Breathe normally and see your heart glowing with a red, fiery light.
6. This practice will strengthen your heart and activate the heart's virtues of love, inner joy, happiness, and sincerity. With each breath you take, try to feel red light replacing the hot, toxic energy of hastiness, hatred, arrogance, and cruelty. As the red fire energy expands in your heart and you cleanse yourself of the negative energies there, good emotional qualities will have room to grow. Feel love, joy, honor, and respect radiating outward. Feel any hatred, arrogance, or impatience becoming transformed into loving energy as sincerity, honor, and respect grow in your heart. Try to maintain those feelings as long as you can after you finish the practice (figure 9.19).
7. Repeat the sequence three to six times. Practice more to relieve sore throats, cold sores, swollen gums, or a swollen tongue, as well as jumpiness, moodiness, and heart disease.

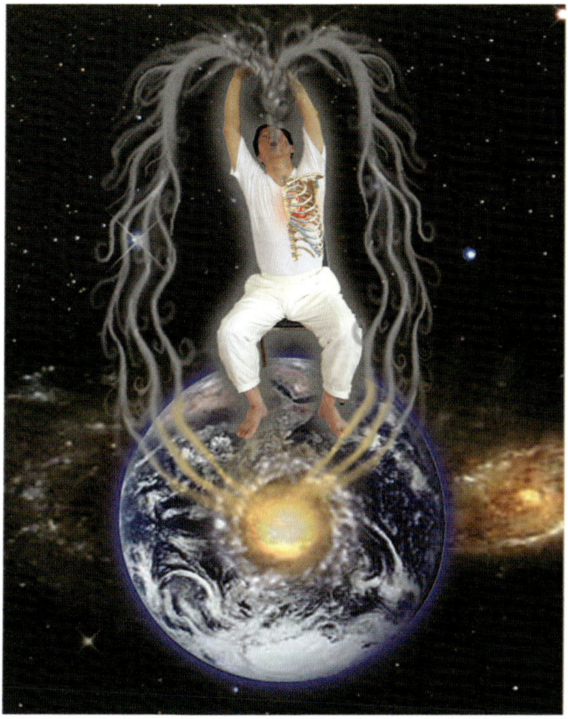

Fig. 9.17. Make the heart sound.

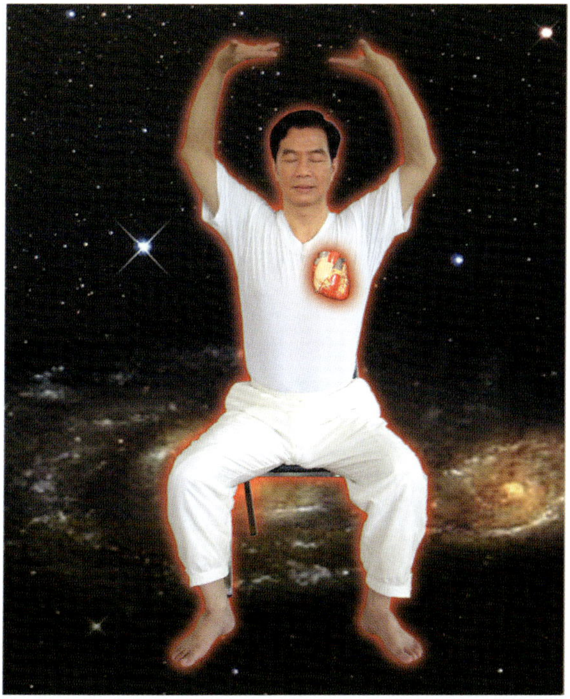

Fig. 9.18. Gather energy to pour into your heart.

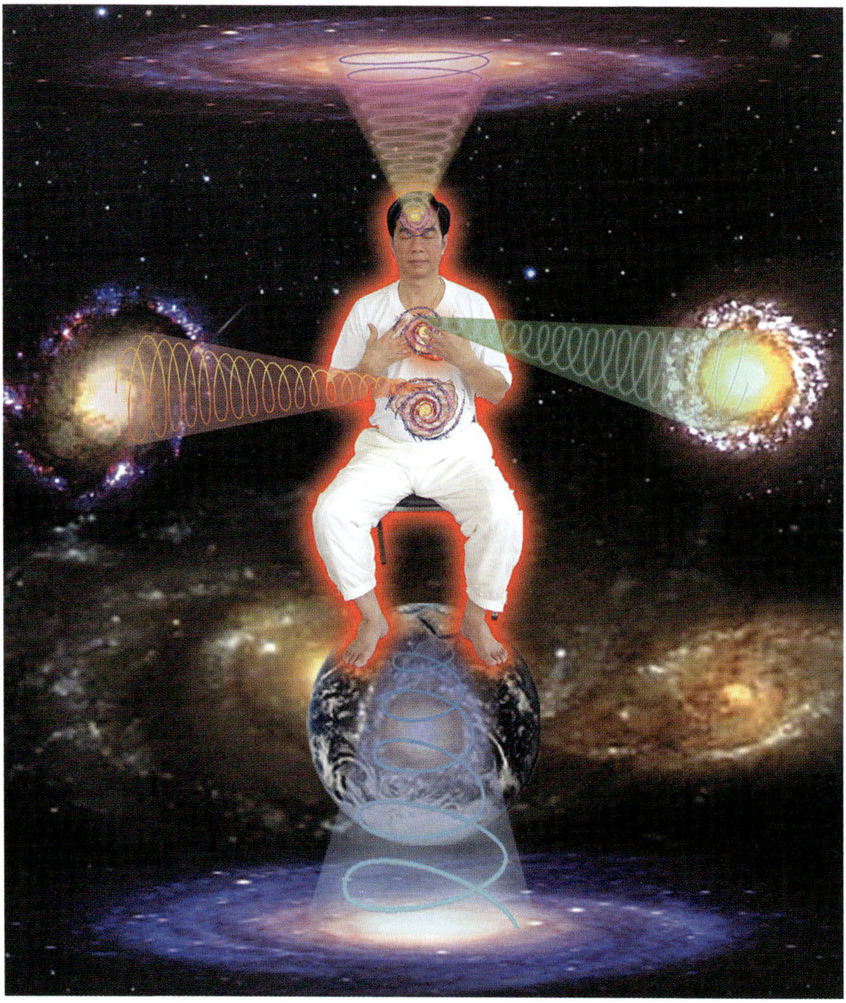

Fig. 9.19. Loving energy grows in your heart when you practice the heart sound.

Spleen Sound: Fifth Healing Sound

The spleen sound is an earth sound that activates the energy of the spleen, pancreas, and stomach.

Associated organs: pancreas and stomach
Element: earth
Season: Indian summer
Color: yellow
Emotions: worry, negative thinking, overthinking
Virtues: openness, fairness, balance, trust
Associated parts of the body: lips, mouth
Sense: taste
Tastes: sweet, neutral
Sound: *whoooooooo*, a guttural sound coming from your throat

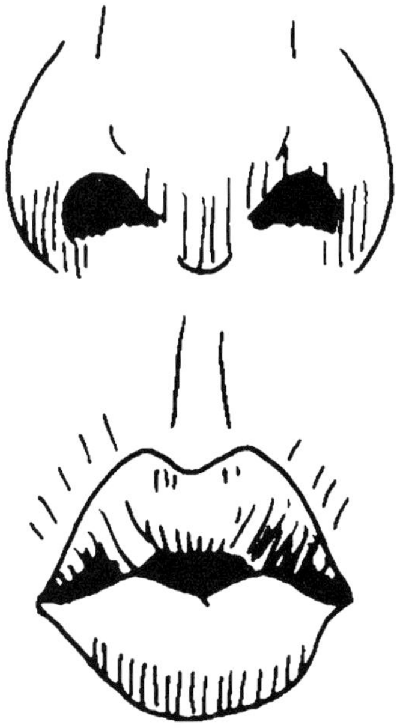

Fig. 9.20. Make the spleen sound with lips rounded and pursed.

1. Sit comfortably on the edge of a chair with your back straight. Rest your palms on your spleen. Close your eyes. Smile down at your stomach and spleen until you can feel that you have connected with them. Notice the quality of energy in your stomach and spleen. Picture a yellow light around your spleen, the golden, satiated light of Indian summer (figure 9.21).
2. Take a deep breath, open your eyes, and move your arms in front of your body. Place the three middle fingers of both hands just below your ribs on the left side of your rib cage. Look up and press your fingers into your body under your rib cage, which pushes your spleen back and pushes the middle of your back outward.
3. Slowly exhale, lean forward, and make the spleen sound, *whoooooooo*. It is a more guttural or throaty sound than the kidney sound. Unlike blowing out a candle, this sound originates in the chest rather than from the mouth. You can make the sound out loud at first. Eventually you will be able to make it subvocally.

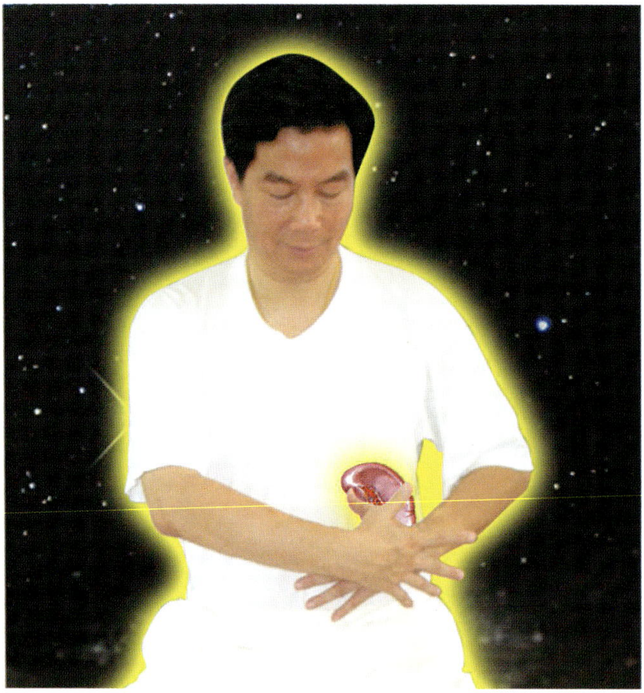

Fig. 9.21. Smile at your spleen.

4. Feel the vibration of the spleen sound start to move the energy in your spleen, pancreas, and stomach. Feel the excess heat and toxins being expelled from them as the sacs around them are compressed (figure 9.22).
5. After you have fully exhaled, slowly sit back up, reach your arms outward, embrace the earth, and scoop up yellow light in your palms. Pour that light into your spleen, pancreas, and stomach. Now bring your palms back to your spleen. Allow the yellow light and the virtues of fairness, openness, and trust to radiate in your spleen, pancreas, and stomach.
6. Rest. Close your eyes, and focus on your stomach, pancreas, and spleen. Smile at them and imagine that you are still making the spleen sound. Feel the vibration of the sound moving and cleaning the energy of those organs.
7. Breathe normally. See your stomach, pancreas, and spleen glowing with a yellow light. This exercise strengthens those organs and

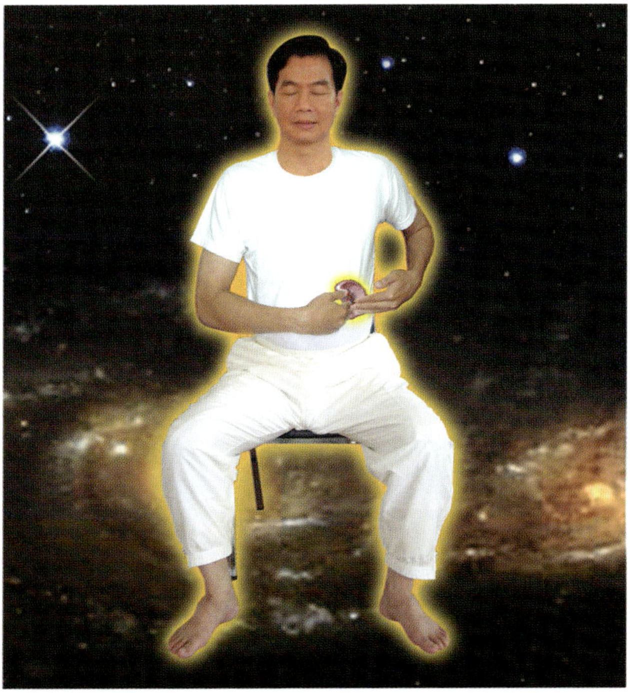

Fig. 9.22.
Press your fingers under your left rib cage.

activates the virtues of fairness, openness, trust, and stability. With each breath you take, try to feel the warm, yellow light replacing hot, toxic energy and worry, negative thinking, and overthinking in the organs.

8. Nurture good emotions. This is the most important part of this practice. Take all the time you need to get in touch with your pancreas, stomach, and spleen. As you rid those organs of excess heat and let the yellow earth energy expand in them, good emotional qualities will have room to grow. Try to maintain the feelings from this exercise as long as you can afterward (figure 9.23).
9. Repeat the sequence three to six times. Practice more to eliminate indigestion, nausea, and diarrhea.

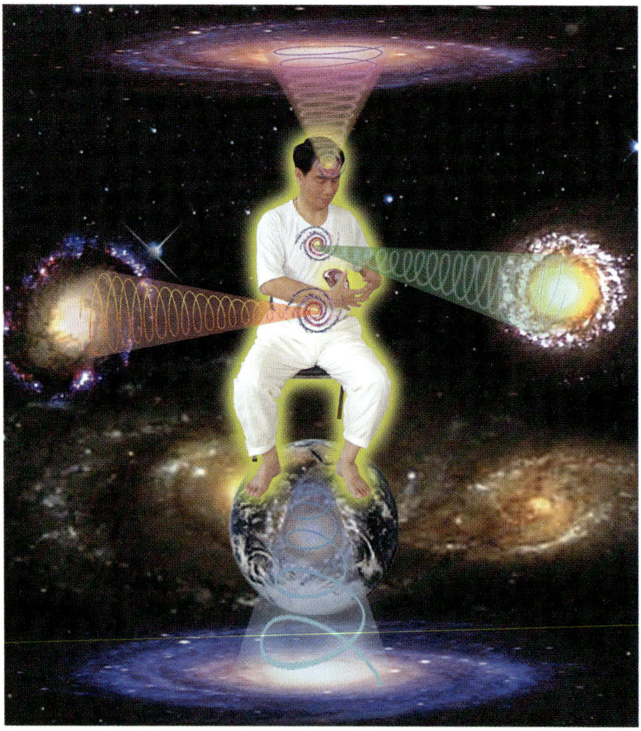

Fig. 9.23. Bring yellow light to your spleen and allow openness and fairness to grow in it.

Triple Warmer Sound: Sixth Healing Sound

The triple warmer refers to the three energy centers in the body and their respective levels of warmth: the upper section, which includes the brain, heart, and lungs, is hot; the middle section, which includes the liver, kidneys, stomach, pancreas, and spleen, is warm; and the lower section, which includes the large and small intestines, bladder, and sexual organs, is cool. The triple warmer sound, *heeeeeeeee*, balances the temperatures of the three levels by bringing hot energy down to the lower center and cool energy up to the higher center (figure 9.24). Specifically, hot energy from the area of the heart is moved to the cool sexual region, and cooler energy from the lower abdomen is moved up to the area of the heart. Note that the triple warmer sound is best done lying down to facilitate falling asleep.

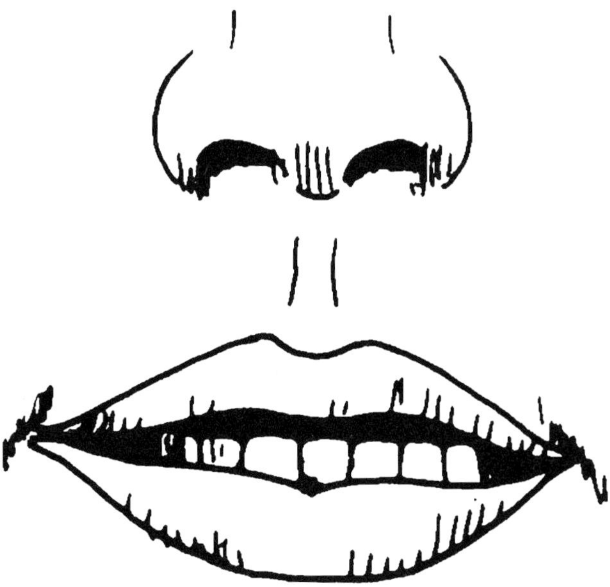

Fig. 9.24. Make the *heeeeeeee* sound while exhaling with the lips.

1. Lie on your back. Smile. Move your arms and hands upward as you scoop up chi. Bring your hands to your face. Exhale slowly and make the triple warmer sound, *heeeeeeee*. As you make the sound, let

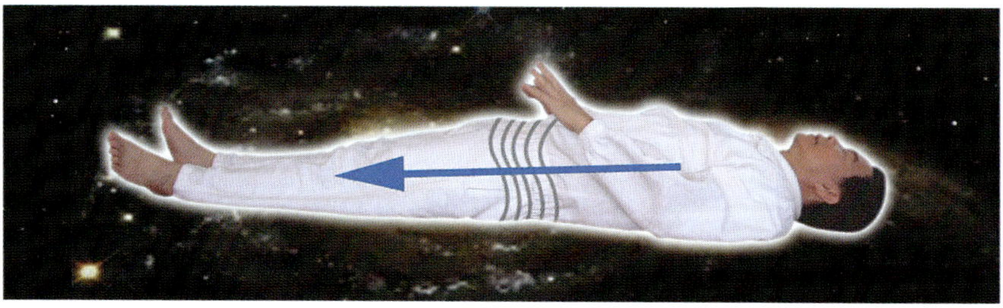

Fig. 9.25. Gather up chi as you raise your arms.

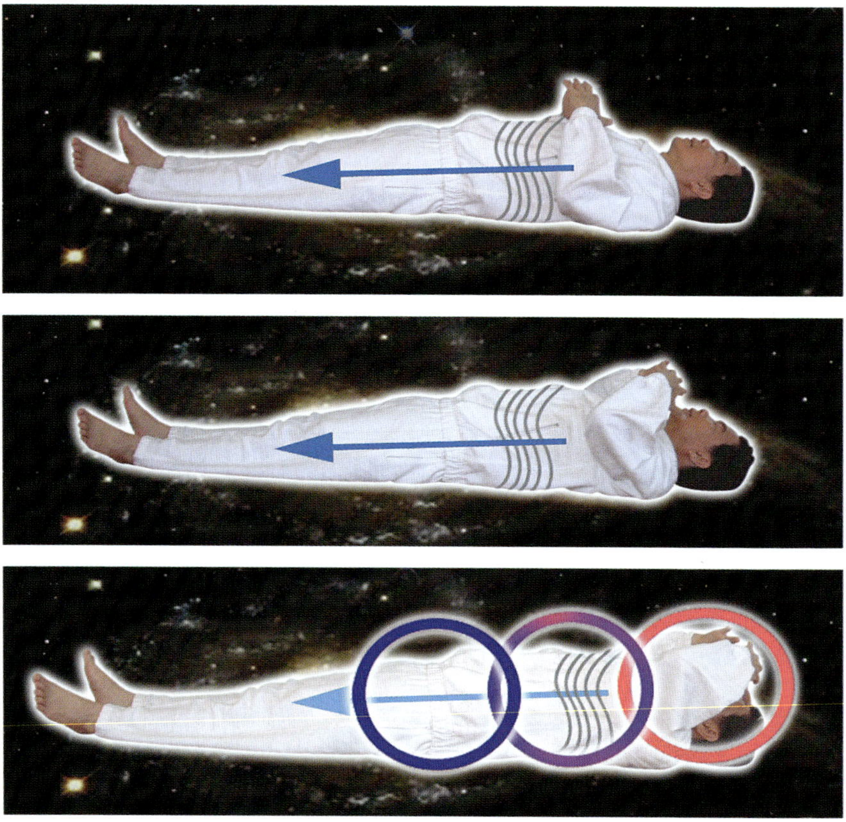

Fig. 9.26. The triple warmer sound moves down the body from the upper level to the middle level and then to the lower level.

your arms move slowly down your body, bringing the energy down from your crown to your feet (figures 9.25 and 9.26).

2. Inhale fully into all three cavities: your chest, solar plexus, and lower abdomen. Then slowly exhale completely while you make the triple

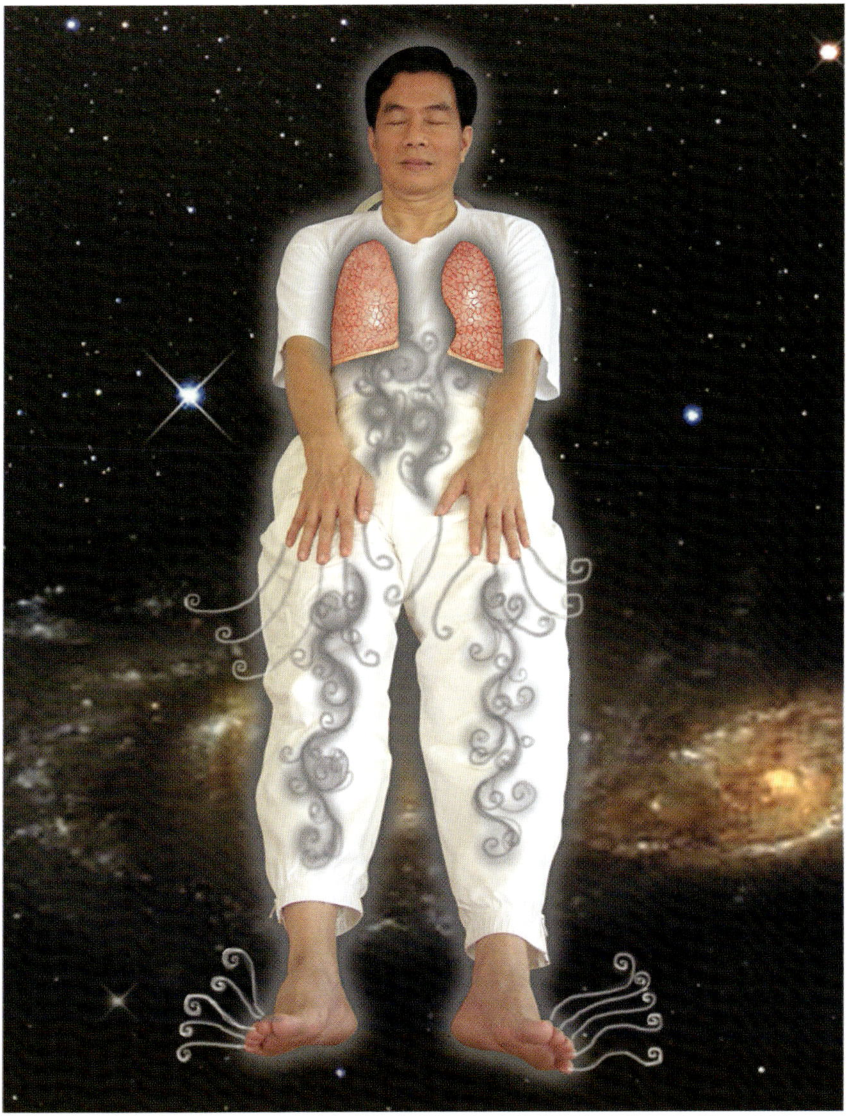

Fig. 9.27. Excess heat flows out of your fingertips and toes and into the earth.

warmer's sound, *heeeeeeee*. You can make the sound out loud when you first start practicing it. Eventually you will be able to make it subvocally. As you exhale and make the sound, flatten your chest, then your solar plexus, and finally your lower abdomen. Imagine a large roller pressing out your breath and moving the hot energy down as your arms move from your head down to your Lower Tan Tien.

3. Now point your fingers at your toes and let excess heat and toxins release out of the tips of your fingers and toes. It goes into the earth to be recycled (figure 9.27).
4. Rest. Focus on your entire digestive tract. Repeat the sequence three six times. Practice more to relieve insomnia and stress.

10

Practices for Releasing Trauma

We all know that some events in our past are easier to let go of than others. Some experiences seem to get stuck inside of us, taking up energetic space. These kinds of traumatic experiences can weigh us down emotionally and block the energy channels in the body, which can lead to physical pain and heightened emotional sensitivity. This is reflected in our language, in such expressions as "It really weighs on me," or "I've had it up to here with that," or "You're working on my last nerve." Now is a good time to remind the reader of an earlier point, which is that the steady pileup of small, unprocessed emotions from everyday life events can eventually carry the same weight as a single traumatic event, with the result being the same—a feeling of a lack of control.

In the case of unprocessed trauma, anytime you encounter something that directly or indirectly connects to that original painful experience, you are triggered to experience its effects on your emotional body again. It takes a lot of energy to keep those unresolved thoughts and feelings connected to traumatic events of the past out of your conscious awareness. As long as the aftereffects of those issues remain unaddressed, they leave you in kind of a "yellow alert" state wherein you are hypervigilant, always bracing for the same old problems to crop up. When this happens, the tendency to want to self-medicate is an automatic reaction. If you have a history of addiction, your system will seek that solution first because it has proven to be somewhat powerful and effective in the past. Even if you are working hard to stay away from your addiction, those thoughts and urges lie dormant and can still be activated. Therefore it is very important to address those deep underlying issues that are associated with some kind of trauma.

TAOIST EMOTIONAL RECYCLING

A technique known as Taoist Emotional Recycling (TER) can be used to neutralize and recycle, and thereby transform, the negative emotions and energies that linger when people have overwhelming experiences that they cannot understand or fix.* We present this technique here in a somewhat abbreviated form because without addressing the pileup of the larger toxic emotional energies held by someone who has struggled with addiction, their recovery is left in a vulnerable state.

There have been many approaches developed over the years that have attempted to help people let go of the negative residue of past experiences in quick, relatively painless, and permanent ways. We believe that TER accomplishes that goal. In this chapter we will outline how to use the technique to address past experiences that linger and still provoke negative emotional reactions in the present. TER was designed to operate in keeping with the principles of Taoism and the Universal Healing Tao system. It is a synthesis of the elements of a Western counseling approach known as EMDR, which stands for

*Most of our book *EMDR and the Universal Healing Tao: An Energy Psychology Approach to Overcoming Emotional Trauma*, was devoted to explaining how the technique that was described in it, Taoist Emotional Recycling (TER), was developed, its connections to Western psychology and Taoist theory and practice, and how to use it correctly.

Eye Movement Desensitization and Reprocessing, along with a few Universal Healing Tao practices. The result of this blending is a technique that produces complete results quickly and often without too much emotional distress.

EMDR has been revolutionary in the counseling field. The eye movement aspect of it presents an opportunity to bridge Western and Eastern practices, and TER is the result. Taoist Chi Kung practitioners and instructors have been using eye movement to create emotional benefits for over five thousand years. Even though EMDR is a powerful tool in its own right, there is always room for experimentation and improvement. This is where TER comes in. This Taoist practice is different than EMDR in several notable ways. As is the case for all of the Universal Healing Tao practices, it is designed to be a self-help tool. It addresses the effects of emotional upset on the body in a much more comprehensive and systematic fashion than EMDR. Since we are working directly with the organs of the body that each create particular emotions, mental states, and spiritual experiences, we have removed some of the standard phases in the EMDR protocol that address those levels of experience separately. The result is that many of the preliminary questions and preparatory exercises are replaced with Universal Healing Tao practices. Different kinds of eye movements have been added to enhance the emotional processing. For example, your eyes are open in EMDR when you process with eye movement; they are closed in TER. EMDR follows the trail of thoughts that occur during the processing and continues from where the person left off in the last set of movements. In TER we use the same initial focus to start each set. Of course, Taoism and Taoist Chi Kung also offer theoretical and philosophical ways to understand how the process works, why people react in the ways they do, and what they need to do if the process is not proceeding smoothly or typically. We gave our process a different name because we changed the procedure so much that it does not look much like EMDR anymore.

Who Should Consider TER?

Very often, trauma is not addressed in various addiction treatment settings due to the amount of time it would take to address it properly, along with the concern that some people might become so triggered that it might actually work against the stability of their recovery. Therefore, the decision about when to start working on those deep underlying issues can be tricky. On the one hand, unresolved trauma can trigger the desire to self-medicate. On the other hand, treating those issues might disturb the person to the point where it stimulates a desire to return to their addiction. It is really important to proceed with caution before deciding to open up old emotional wounds. The experiences that you have had with the other exercises in this book can give you a clue about how ready your system is for this next level of healing. If you have experienced negative emotions, nightmares, or a sense of being out of touch with the current moment, or you feel like your experiences are not real or feel numb when you have tried any of the other practices, then it is advisable to wait to address your deep underlying trauma until that stops happening. Emotional healing is not a "no pain, no gain" proposition. Do not try to be tough and push through no matter what. That will only produce more overwhelming feelings and more toxic buildup as a result. Keep in mind that the other exercises in this book also address the buildup of toxic energies in your life, just in more indirect and gentler ways than TER. Flowing water can erode solid rock, given enough time. If you start going through the TER process and you end up with any of those adverse reactions, stop the process and return to the earlier practices that help you calm down and reconnect with the present moment. The Six Healing Sounds is a very good practice if that's the case.

If you are certain that you are ready to start addressing the weight of events from your past using TER, the first task is to identify the unresolved emotions that need to be addressed. In other words, what is the specific issue that you want to address? The issue could be very general at first. The focus will be narrowed down later in the process. For example, some people at first will know only that they have unresolved issues with how they were raised. Others might know that they have trouble saying "no" when they need to, and that has caused problems for them. Other people might have identified issues that are generally recognized as potentially having traumatic consequences, such as going to war, being in a car accident, and experiencing any kind of abuse.

If you feel ready you may choose to address a particular trigger that threatens to take you back to active addiction. It could be a person, place, thing, or situation. Keep in mind that triggers can be negative or positive. Sometimes people are reluctant to acknowledge or accept that there is still a part of them that longs for the positive effects that their addiction used to provide—when you think about it, if there were no positive experiences associated with it, then you wouldn't have continued to use whatever it is that you were addicted to. If you are trying to stay away from an addiction, it is also important to recognize that you will not be able to remove those memories, but you can neutralize their pull on you. Leaving a positive trigger like that unrecognized or untreated could be as dangerous as a negative trigger. Positive triggers are experiences that were experienced as generally positive at the time, and encourage a person to try to repeat that experience when they are activated, even if repeating the experience could be harmful or dangerous. Many people have positive experiences when they first try drugs like cocaine, for example. Even though they may realize later that they should abstain from using cocaine, a deeper, automatic urge to feel the way they did with initial experimentation can linger and threaten to derail their recovery. In 12-Step meetings, participants are warned about the dangers of "romancing the addiction," as they put it. This reflects an awareness of the dangers of such positive triggers.

Usually when we think about things that need healing, we search our memories for instances of abuse of some kind or an overwhelming event like war or surviving a tsunami. Of course, those kinds of events are legitimate for this process. However, a legitimate issue might only register a 2 on a scale of 0 to 10 in terms of emotional severity. If it happened a long time ago and it still brings up emotions when you think about it, then it is worth addressing. Do you know the folktale of the Princess and the Pea? The gist of the story is that the princess cannot sleep because there is one pea under her mattress. She doesn't know it's there, so she tries to make the bed more comfortable on top. She cannot sleep until the pea is found and removed. If you do not know that story, maybe you have had the experience of trying to sleep but there is a fly or a mosquito buzzing around in your room. It's worthwhile to address anything and everything in your personal history that disturbs your peace. You may also be aware that some of your emotional remnants are due to seeing someone else go through something that was difficult or painful in some way, such as experiencing the effects of war up close or seeing one parent abuse the other parent. Do not minimize or ignore those kinds of traumas. Sometimes the witness is even more affected by an event than the person who was directly involved.

Shame is a particular negative trigger that almost always has to be addressed in recovery. Even if a person understands intellectually that what they did during active addiction was out of character and not done when the person was in her or his right mind, that does not necessarily heal the negative feelings around what happened. Then too, neglect is often overlooked as a potential issue, but it can have a big impact on how people see themselves, their self-worth, and what they are capable of in life. It can be an irrational belief that a person carries about him- or herself. The person may not experience that belief on a conscious level and may already know that it is not actually true, but that does not guarantee that the belief does not still limit the person. A single belief can negatively affect so many aspects of daily living. The original EMDR protocol did an excellent job of identifying those beliefs. Examples of irrational negative beliefs are "I am bad," "I am dirty," "I am not loveable," "I do not deserve," and "It's my fault." The issue might even be a pattern of behavior that you really want to change or a pattern of undesirable results that you want to discontinue.

Sometimes people struggle with where to start. They can identify so many issues that it's difficult to decide which one they should address first. You can make that choice based on any criteria you choose. You might want to identify the first event that you can remember that affected your life in a negative way. Maybe you want to choose the biggest obstacle first. Maybe you want to address the most recent issue because it is the one that is foremost on your mind. Perhaps you prefer to start with a small issue and get used to the process before moving on to a bigger one. Keep in mind, though, that your perception of what carries the most and least emotional charge might change once you start the TER process. For example, sometimes the issue you choose may seem minor, but once you start unearthing all of the unconscious connections to it in your mind, you end up feeling more agitated than you anticipated. Some people agonize over finding the root issue to their problems. Usually there is no one thing, though; there will be a bunch of issues that have not been resolved. Try not to spend too much time and energy looking for that one brick in the wall that will bring the whole thing tumbling down if you pull it out. Remember that you are learning how to use this approach, and you can use it as many times as you like, so in a sense it is not so important which issue you address first. As long as you keep using the technique, you will eventually address all of them.

The next task is to identify what you will focus on to start the process, combing through your memories to find the issue, something like using a search term on the internet to find the right file. Usually this will be a visual memory, but it can also be a memory from any other sense as long as it produces a reaction inside of you that you want to remove. A visual is preferred because it has so much information in it that it makes for a good search term. However, sometimes a visual is not what stands out for a person. It may instead be the sound of a voice that you can still hear ringing in your ears. It could be a certain smell. It could even be a certain feeling in your body. Whatever you choose to focus on, make sure it is a real experience that you have had in connection with the issue. In other words, if your focus is a visual image, you should not be able to see yourself in that picture unless you were looking at an actual photo that was taken with a camera or you were floating above your body in a near-death experience. When you suffer trauma, your eyes will project outward. What you see at the time of the event does not include you. If your logical mind tells you that creating a picture better represents the issue than your memories can provide, do not listen to your logic. If you use a fictional memory as your search term, then you will access a created file rather than the real experience, and the processing will not work. Neglect is a tricky matter to focus on in this process because it refers to the absence of something. Instead, focus on a common area in your home to access feelings of neglect, like your living room or kitchen table, and go from there.

For the sake of monitoring your progress as you work on the issue, take note of the intensity of your reaction to the narrowed focus that you are using as a search term when you start processing. Check it along the way. It may change rather than decrease at times. That is still progress. Do not move on to another body area in the process until you have completely neutralized your reaction in the body area that you are currently addressing.

HOW TO MAKE THE MOST OF TER

Before you begin TER, there are a number of tips to follow to make the process more effective and more manageable:

- **Choose your own issue or issues to address.** Someone you trust can have some input in your process but avoid addressing issues simply because someone else thinks that is your problem or because you *think* you should address them.
- **Commit to wanting to completely neutralize the impact of that issue before you start.** It is natural to have some hesitation about letting it go, especially if you have carried that issue inside of you for a long time. We tend to make friends with our pain over time, even identifying with it. You may be concerned about how it might feel or what you'll be like after you let such a big thing go. This feeling is natural—know that you will be the same person, minus some unnecessary baggage that robs you of your ability to fully enjoy life. You will still think the same as before. Deciding that it is time to move on from that issue will likely reduce the amount of time you will have to spend on an emotional rollercoaster as you work through the issue.
- **Forgiveness, including self-forgiveness, is not required to go through this process.** Sometimes people struggle with the notion of forgiveness because the issue they are addressing is not something that should be excused. Remember that your opinions and thoughts about the issue will remain after the process is complete. The objective is to neutralize the reactions that are preventing you from moving on with your life.
- **Create a relaxing environment for yourself and take time to relax before you begin.** If you are halfway to the boiling point before you even start, then it will not take much for you to

become overwhelmed by the process. We are trying to remove overwhelming feelings, not add to them.

- **Give yourself permission to proceed at whatever pace works best for you.** There is no deadline in this process. You will not lose the progress you gained if you stop and start over again later. In a counseling session, a person might work consistently for an hour or more at a time. For some people that is exhausting. Even if you only worked on an issue for a few minutes each day, eventually that will add up to a lot of healing.
- **Be aware that even though you are only moving your eyes, the process can be very draining.** On the interior there is a lot happening to produce the healing that comes from doing TER. Check your energy level frequently along the way. Err on the side of caution. If you start to feel even a bit tired, stop for a while or completely. If you feel even more tired after you stop, that is common. If you take it easy for the rest of the day you will usually be back to your normal energy level by the next day.
- **Your eyes can get sore along the way.** To do TER you will be moving your eyes in ways that you normally do not, and more than you normally do as well. If your eyes start to get sore, then between sets of eye movements you can close your eyes and gently rub them, especially along the edges of your eye sockets, to soothe them and loosen up the muscles that are being used to make the eye movements.
- **The process is a healing meditation.** It is supposed to be performed in a relaxed fashion. If you are working really hard to make something happen, you are probably trying too hard. The process is natural. Even if what happens does not make sense to you, try to just play along with the steps of the procedure and trust that whatever happens is what's needed for the healing to happen.
- **The process is not enhanced if you concentrate harder or try to focus on particular aspects of the experience.** You do not

need to have clear images in your mind before you begin the process. You do not have to hold more than one focus at a time. You do not need to hold onto your search term throughout the processing. Think about a streaming video. If you want to watch a show but you keep dragging it back to the beginning, you will never finish that show. Just let it play out.

- **The most typical reaction in the process is that over time the beginning image that people have been using to start the process starts to fade, then parts of it start to disappear or it starts to slide down their field of vision, or it just becomes difficult to focus on it.** That's a good sign! It becomes difficult to react to the image if you can no longer see it clearly. If something like that happens to you, take comfort in knowing that it happens to almost everyone who experiences TER.
- **Sometimes people worry when they do not get a negative reaction when they start to work on an issue in a new area of their body.** This process is like an archeological dig: you cannot know ahead of time where you will find reactions. If you do not react, that is not a bad thing. Complaining about that would be like complaining that you found a bedroom that is already clean when you are vacuuming the rooms in your home. Why would you complain about that? Be grateful for that and move on.
- **During the processing there is a natural tendency to explain away when you have reactions in other parts of your body than in the area you are focused on.** For example, you may have a reaction in your back when you are processing, even though that is not where you are focusing during the processing. It would be easy to conclude that you are just sitting in an awkward position, that you have been sitting for too long, or something like that. Remember, though, in TER we are working with the meridians, the energy channels that thread throughout the body from the organs that we are addressing in TER. As a result, you could

have an unexpected reaction in your body because the energy that has been stimulated and flushed through those channels has produced a reaction along one of those pathways. If you feel a unexpected reaction like that, assume that the processing in the area you are focused on is not finished yet and do it again.

- **Everyone responds in their own unique ways to the processing.** Over time you will probably start to notice patterns in how you respond to the process. In the meantime, assume that whatever happens is what's needed for you. Some people feel strongly at times. Others never feel like that. Some people have thoughts along the way. Others do not. The most common experience, however, is that whatever someone expects to happen is not what happens.
- **Do not be discouraged if you have difficulty moving your eyes in the ways that are described in this approach.** When you first start addressing an issue, it is common to have trouble performing the eye movements. The reason is that the emotion surrounding the issue you are addressing is thick inside you, so your eyes feel like they are dredging through mud when you try to move them. Smooth, easy eye movements do not produce better results than jerky, sputtering ones. Sometimes your eyes may do something completely different than what you are trying to make them do. Trust that it must be what you need and just go along with the experience.
- **The more issues you address using TER, the faster they tend to be able to be addressed.** Picture a room filled to the ceiling with boxes. Getting the first couple of boxes out could be difficult, but once you have those out it is easier to move around in the space and get the rest of them out.
- **Often the next issue presents itself automatically right after you finish the one you are currently addressing.** Your mind seems to operate in a similar way to those shelves in a supermar-

ket that have rollers on them: once you pull the item at the front of the shelf off, the next item automatically rolls to the front.

- **If moving your eyes is not workable for you, you can use your hands instead.** Place one palm on the body area you are going to work on so that your palm is on that part. Then put the other palm on top of it. Move the two palms together in the same direction that you would otherwise move your eyes in the exercise. If you want an even more intense experience, move your hands and eyes at the same time. This is not required, and it takes more concentration, so it may be quite a while before you attempt that.
- **Notice that the emotional reactions in each body area that you are addressing fit with the emotional reactions associated with that area.** They often match exactly. There is a reason why Taoists have been connecting certain emotions to certain organs for over five thousand years. Let yourself have the experience first before you check to see if they match the theoretical connections in each area. Then you will not have to wonder afterward if you only had those reactions because you had an expectation based on what you read prior to going through the process.
- **If you feel dizzy or nauseous during the processing of your issue, you are probably moving your eyes or hands too quickly.** Faster movements do not lead to better results. Slow down. Think about trying to clean up a table that has a lot of little things piled on top of it. Moving too quickly can make more of a mess. Drink some water and take time to make sure you are breathing from your abdomen before continuing the process.
- **Do not count how many times you move your eyes or palms in a certain way when you are doing TER.** If you do that it will be difficult to concentrate on anything else, and it might interfere with your ability to naturally work through the issue. An approximate number of movements will work fine. You are just

trying to move energy and recycle the unprocessed material in each area. Think about a sink full of water that someone has just used to wash their face. How many times does that person need to swish the water before any soap foam in it has dispersed? No one knows. An exact number of movements does not guarantee anything.

- **Each movement of your eyes and/or hands should take approximately two seconds.**
- **Make sure you have tissues and water nearby before you start in case you need them.**
- **You do not have to process each picture or sensory memory of the issue that you are addressing one at a time.** The processing works on much more than the aspect that you are focusing on at the beginning. We are just using that like a search term to get the associated file. Then the eye and/or hand movements will work on the whole file. Otherwise it would take far too long to heal from your past trauma. The proof will be at the end of the process: you will notice that you do not react to many (maybe all) aspects of the issue, not just the part that you used to start the process. If some part of the issue still bothers you after you complete the exercise (which does not happen often), then take a new focal point out of that remaining portion and go through the process again, using that new focal point as your starting point.
- **Measuring progress with an approach like this can be tricky because when it works, you will just feel nothing and/or normal.** If you are working on an issue over several days, progress will be noticeable more in terms of degree. You may feel less upset about the issue when you think about it or talk about it. You might have the issue come to mind less often. It might take less time or effort to regain your composure when it comes to mind again.

- **Always check to make sure the issue is completely processed in an area before you move on to the next one.** Use the methods for checking that are offered in this chapter. You may feel very certain that the issue is completely neutralized in an area, but keep in mind that you probably were not aware of how much your mind and body were affected by the issue until you started this process. Some effects of the issue are deeply buried. They are like weeds in the sense that if you leave some piece of it behind, it may grow back into something big later. So be thorough.
- **Notice that positive emotions, thoughts, and beliefs about yourself tend to increase naturally the more you do the TER process.** Remember that this is a recycling process. Energy cannot be created or destroyed, but it can be transformed. We are recycling your old emotional, mental, physical and spiritual garbage into healthier, happier energy. Another way to think about the process is that as old, heavy, dense, negative energy is processed into lighter, brighter energy, more space is created inside of you. That leaves more room for positive thoughts, feelings, and beliefs to grow.
- **When you want to get rid of a file in a computer, first you delete the file and send it to the trash bin, then you empty the trash bin to recycle.** In theory, as you move your eyes and/or hands from side to side, it is producing a response inside of you that is comparable to the delete function in a computer. It is not deleting in the sense of destroying energy. That is impossible. It is deleting the connections between the various bits of information about that issue that are clumped inside of you. The spiraling movements are comparable to the recycle function of a computer. You gather the connections to the issue or file and then compact them into the smallest space possible.

Processing Trauma in Your Center of Happiness

We begin with the Center of Happiness, located in the upper mind just behind the middle of your forehead:

1. Sit erect on the edge of a chair and place your feet flat on the floor. Smile.
2. Close your eyes and focus on the middle of your forehead. Mentally place the chosen issue (your "search term") in the middle of your forehead.
3. Move your eyes and/or hands left and right, looking left and right inside your brain. Do that for about eighteen sets. One set consists of moving your eyes or palms to the left and to the right once each time.
4. Now, with your eyes still closed, slowly make spiral movements with your eyes and/or palms while continuing to focus on the issue in the middle of your forehead. Make small circles that become progressively larger. Make approximately eighteen spirals.
5. Now reverse the direction of the spiraling and make circles that get progressively smaller for approximately twelve revolutions.
6. Rest for a minute as you open your eyes and take your mind off the issue. Once you feel rested and ready, repeat steps 3–5 consisting of the side-to-side and spiraling movements. Use the same starting point to focus on (your "search term," usually an image) each time you start a new set.
7. Rest between each set of movements. Remember, this process can be surprisingly draining, so pace yourself. Continue each set of repetitions until you no longer feel any negative reaction in the middle of your forehead when you focus on your beginning image, sound, smell, or feeling. After you complete a set of eye and/or hand movements and you suspect that the issue might be completely neutralized in your Center of Happiness, close your eyes and put the

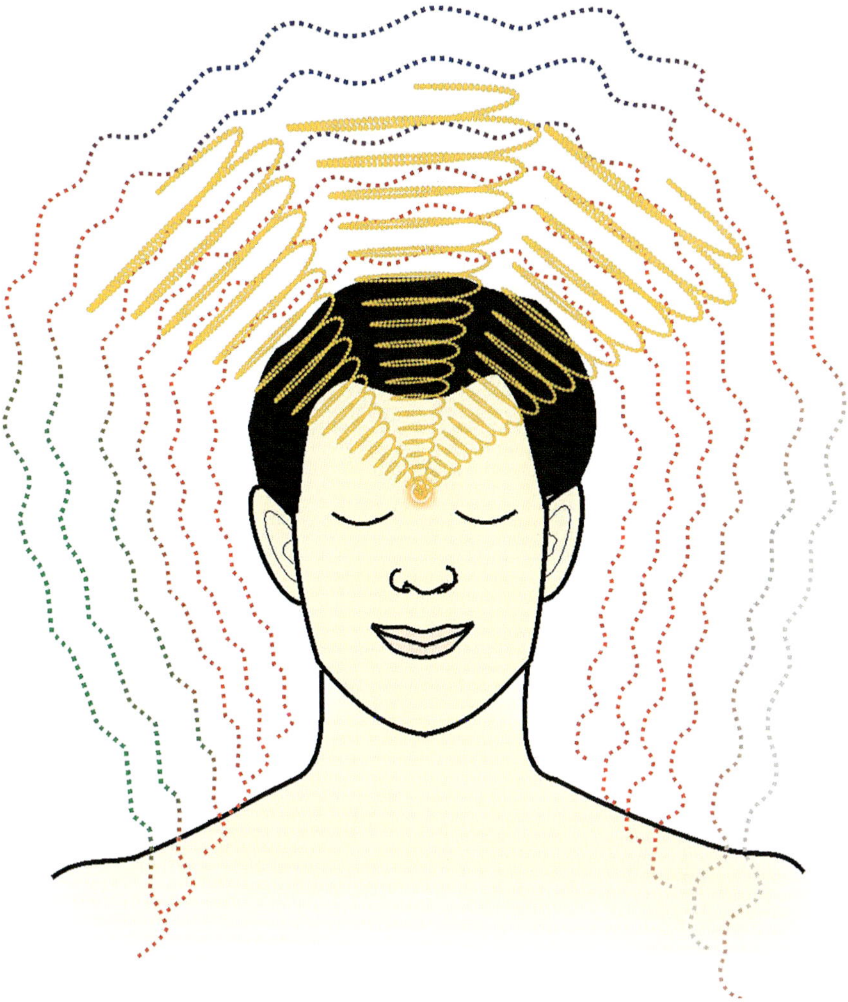

Fig. 10.1. Processing in your Center of Happiness.

starting point back in the middle of your forehead again. This time do not move your eyes. Just focus on it and notice if you feel any kind of negative reaction when you do that. If there are no mind or body reactions to the starting point, then you can move on to the next body area to be processed.

8. If you become too emotional or feel too much heat in your head during the processing, stop and make the lung sound, *ssssssssss*, two

or three times until you feel cool and calm before you proceed. Using the lung sound a few times is an effective way to circulate cool, clean air through your whole body and help you to calm down.

Processing in Your Center of Peace

We will next move to the Center of Peace, located in the heart area:

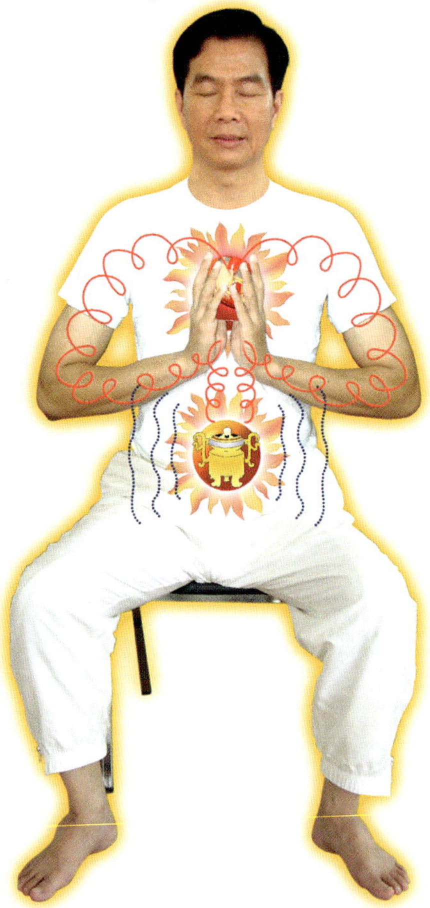

Fig. 10.2. Activate and transform your Center of Peace.

1. Continue to use the same starting point, the issue that you used when you cleared the associated emotions out of your Center of Happiness.
2. Close your eyes. Smile and focus on your heart. See it inside your body. Place your hands on your heart if that helps you to focus there. See the color red around your heart. At first the red color may be dark, cloudy, or murky. As you continue to focus on and smile at your heart, it will become a clearer and brighter red. The darkness in the red is toxic energy, energy that is out of balance. As you smile at it, you transform toxic energy into healthy, virtuous energy. You are transforming hastiness, arrogance, impatience, hatred, and cruelty into joy, happiness, and love.
3. Keep smiling at your heart until the red color does not get any clearer or brighter.
4. Now put your starting point inside of or on top of your heart.
5. Move your eyes and/or hands from side to side for approximately eighteen rotations.
6. Spiral your eyes and/or hands, making circles that become progressively larger, for approximately eighteen sets.
7. Now reverse the direction of the spiraling and make circles that get progressively smaller for approximately twelve rotations.
8. Open your eyes. Rest for a minute. Take your mind off of the issue. Then repeat the side-to-side and spiraling movements. Use the same starting point for each set.
9. Rest. Continue the sets of side-to-side and spiraling movements until you no longer feel any negative reaction in your mind or in your heart when you stop, close your eyes, and focus on your starting point in your heart.
10. If you feel yourself getting too upset during the processing, stop and use the healing sound for the heart, *hawwwwww*, to cool your heart down and keep yourself calm.

Dissolving the Connection between Your Center of Peace and Your Center of Happiness

Residue from the processing that occurs in your organs can float up to your brain, your Center of Happiness, via the vagus nerves, the main nerves of the parasympathetic nervous system that run throughout the body. We want to make sure that all of that residual energy is processed as well. After the reactions in each organ have been processed, we will go back to your forehead and do one set of eye and/or hand movements to accomplish that. One set consists of movements from side to side and both types of spirals. We just finished processing in the heart, so we can do that now:

1. Close your eyes. Smile.
2. Put your starting memory back in the middle of your forehead.
3. Move your eyes and/or hands from side to side for about eighteen sets. Then make little circles getting bigger for about eighteen revolutions. Then change direction and make circles getting smaller for about twelve sets.
4. Rest.

Processing in Your Spleen

1. Move your hands to the far-left side of the front of your body under your ribs, where your spleen is located. Place one palm on top of the other and then place both hands palm side down on your spleen. Smile and focus on your spleen. Try to see it inside your body.
2. See the color yellow around your spleen. As you smile at your spleen, you are transforming toxic energy into virtuous energy. You are transforming worry, negative thinking, and overthinking into the spleen's virtues of openness and trust. Smiling at your spleen will allow any cloudiness in it to become clearer and brighter.

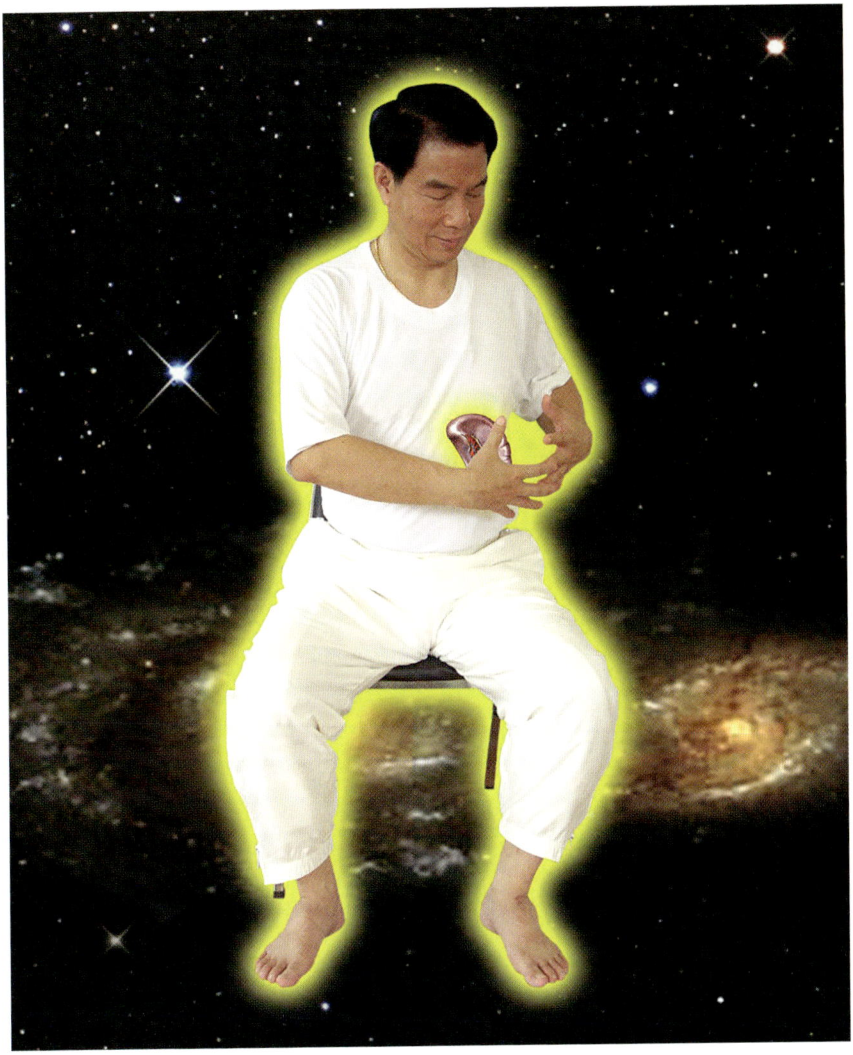

Fig. 10.3. Neutralize the issue in your spleen.

3. Keep smiling at your spleen until the yellow color is completely clear and clean. Then mentally place the issue that you initially chose on top of your spleen.
4. Now close your eyes and move them and/or your hands from side to side for about eighteen sets. Then make spiral movements with little circles getting bigger and bigger for about eighteen sets.

Reverse the direction of your spirals and make big circles that get smaller and smaller for about twelve sets.

5. Rest for a minute. Take your mind off the issue. Then repeat the set movements, starting with the same beginning focus each time, until you no longer feel any reaction during the processing.
6. After you complete a set of movements and you think the issue might be neutralized in your spleen, close your eyes and put the starting focus that you have been using back on your spleen. Focus on it. If you do not feel any reaction to your issue there, then it has been fully addressed in your spleen. You do not have to do any more movements to address that issue there. If you feel the issue is still active, continue with additional sets of movements until you no longer feel a reaction to your issue there.
7. Remember to use the healing sound for the spleen, *whooooooo*, to calm down and cool off your spleen as you work on your issue.

Dissolve the Connection between your Center of Happiness and Your Spleen

Now go back to your forehead and use the back-and-forth and spiraling movements to clear any residual reactions that have moved from your spleen to your brain. You will be moving your eyes and/or hands from side to side for about eighteen sets, then make little circles getting bigger for about eighteen revolutions and then change direction and make circles getting smaller for about twelve sets. You will be repeating this pattern of processing for each organ that follows.

Processing in Your Lungs

1. Place one palm on each of your lungs. Smile at your lungs. Look inside and see your lungs. See white around your lungs. Do not be alarmed if the white color looks dark, cloudy, or murky. The dark-

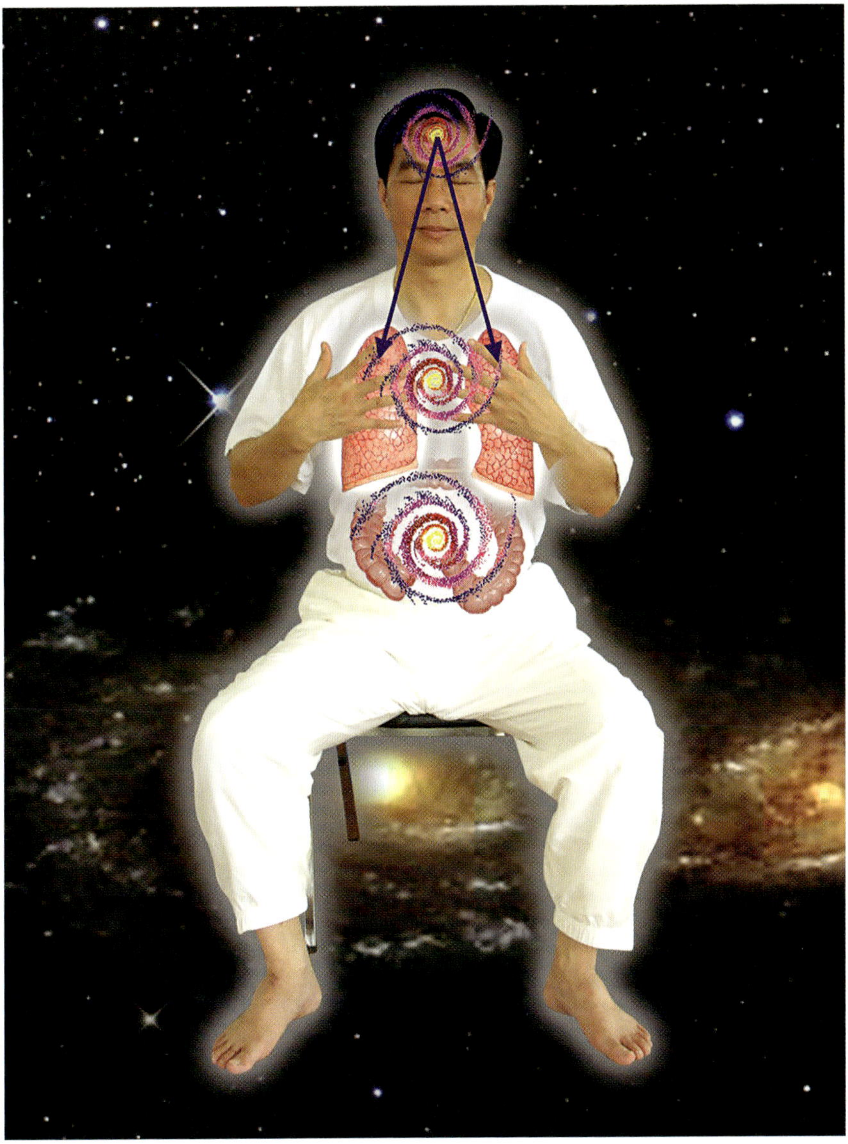

Fig. 10.4. Transform the issue in your lungs.

ness is just toxic energy that you will transform into virtuous energy. As you smile at your lungs you will transform the toxic emotions of grief, sadness, loss, and depression into the lungs' virtues of courage and righteousness.

2. Once you have transformed as much of that toxic energy as possible with the power of your focused smiling energy, mentally place the issue that you chose initially on top of or inside of your lungs.
3. Close your eyes and move your eyes and/or hands from side to side for about eighteen sets. Then make little circles getting bigger and bigger for about eighteen sets. Then reverse the direction of the spirals and make big circles getting smaller and smaller for about twelve sets. Rest.
4. Continue the sets of repetitions until you no longer feel any reaction when you are doing the processing. After you complete a set of eye and/or hand movements and you think the issue might be neutralized in your lungs, close your eyes, focus on your lungs, and put the starting focus back on or in your lungs. If you do not feel a reaction when you do that, then your lungs do not require further processing.
5. To keep your lungs cool and keep yourself calm while processing, use the healing sound for your lungs, *sssssssss*, at any point.

Dissolve the Connection between your Center of Happiness and Your Lungs

Now return once again to your forehead and process the issue out of the area as you have before, with one set of back-and-forth movements of the eyes and one set of spiral movements (eighteen little circles getting bigger and twelve big circles getting smaller). Rest.

Processing in Your Kidneys

1. Smile. Focus on your kidneys. Place one palm on each kidney to make a connection with them. See them inside your body. See the color blue around your kidneys. The blue may not be completely clear and bright at first, but as you smile at your kidneys it will

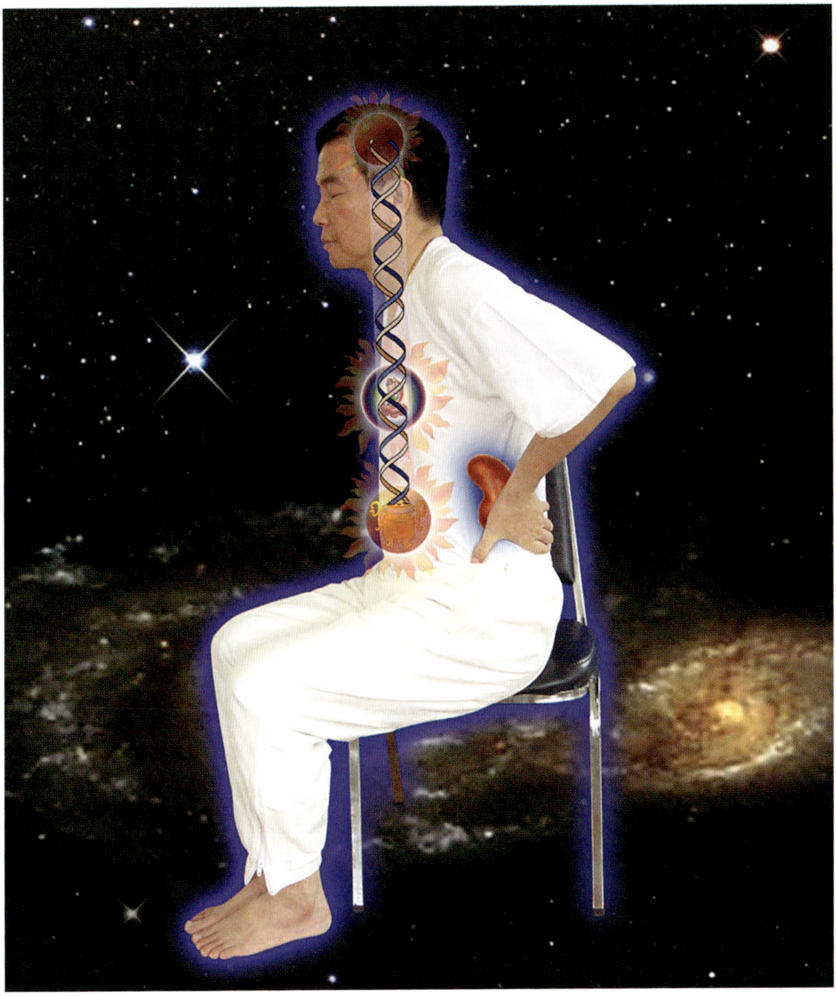

Fig. 10.5. Process negative emotions out of your kidneys.

improve. As you smile at your kidneys you are transforming toxic emotions like fear, guilt, stress, and anxiety into the kidneys' virtues of gentleness, calmness, and stillness. Your willpower increases the more you clean out, balance, and energize your kidneys.

2. When the blue color has brightened and cleared all that it can with the power of your inner smile, focus on the issue you have chosen and mentally place it in or on either of your kidneys.

3. Close your eyes and move them and/or your hands from side to side for about eighteen sets. Then make spiral movements with them, making circles that get bigger and bigger for about eighteen sets. Then reverse the direction of the spirals and make big circles that get smaller and smaller for about twelve sets.
4. Rest for a minute. Take your mind off of the issue. Then repeat the sets of the movements, starting with the same memory each time, until you no longer feel a reaction during the processing.
5. After you complete a set of eye and/or hand movements and you think the issue might be completely neutralized in your kidneys, close your eyes and put the starting memory back on or in your kidneys. If you do not react when you do that, then your kidneys do not need more processing of that issue.

Dissolve the Connection between your Kidneys and Your Center of Happiness

Now return to your forehead and process the issue out of that area in the same manner that you have done before for one set of eye and/or hand movements and spiral movements.

Processing in Your Sexual Organs

1. Place one palm on top of the other and place both palms on your sexual organs. Smile at your sexual organs. See the color pink around them. As you smile at them the pink color will become clearer and brighter. You are restoring the sexual organs' virtues of creativity and vitality.
2. Once the pink color has become as clear and bright as possible from smiling at your sexual organs, mentally place your chosen issue on or in them. Do not be concerned if the issue that you are working on is not of a sexual nature. We are working in this area because we

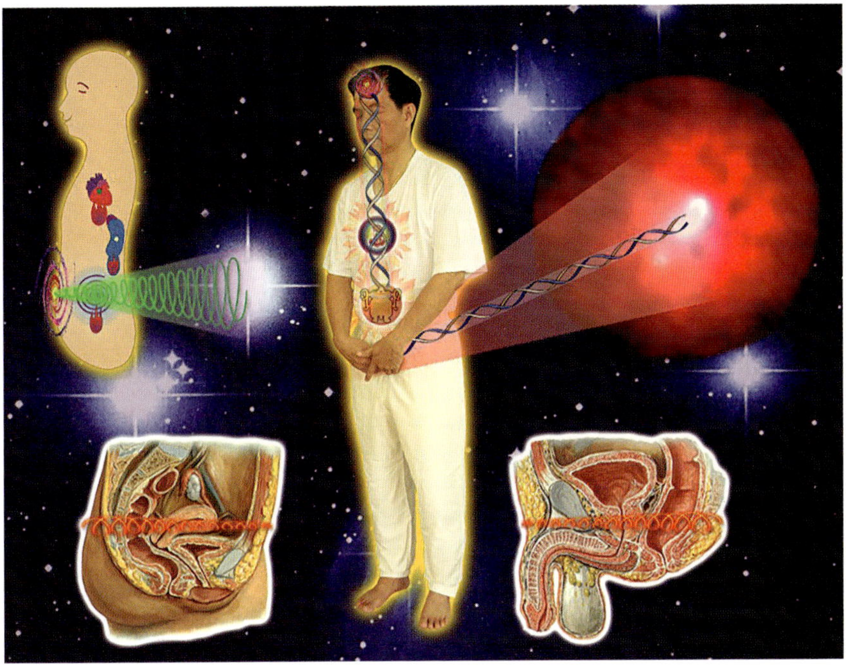

Fig. 10.6. Rebalancing and purifying the energy in your sexual organs.

want to neutralize any emotional content that is coming from your sexual organs that has been affected by the issue.

3. Now close your eyes, smile, and move your eyes and/or hands from side to side for about eighteen sets. Then make spiral motions, making little circles that get bigger and bigger for about eighteen sets. Then reverse the direction of your spirals and make big circles that get smaller and smaller for about twelve sets.
4. Rest for a minute. Take your mind off of the issue. Then resume doing sets of the movements, starting with the same memory each time, until you do not react during the processing.
5. After you complete a set of eye and/or hand movements and you think the issue might be neutralized in your sexual organs, close your eyes and put the memory back in or on your sexual organs. If you do not react when you do that, then the energy in your sexual

organs has been neutralized with regard to your issue. You do not need to do more processing in that area.

Dissolve the Connection between your Sexual Organs and Center of Happiness

Now return to your forehead, smile, and put the memory in the middle of it. Process any residual energy in your Center of Happiness that may be left over from processing in your sexual organs. Do one set of the eye and/or hand movements. Remember to do all of the movements—side-to-side and spiraling movements in each direction.

Processing in Your Liver

1. Your liver is a big triangular-shaped organ on the right side of your body, mostly under your ribs. Place one palm on top of the other and place both hands palms-down on your liver. Smile at your liver. See it inside you. See the color green around it. As you smile at your liver you are transforming the toxic energy inside of it. You are transforming anger, frustration, jealousy, envy, and resentment into the liver's virtues of generosity and kindness. Watch the green color become brighter and clearer as you smile at your liver. Keep doing that until the green color around your liver is as bright and clear as it can be.
2. Close your eyes. Smile. Focus on the issue that you have chosen and mentally place it inside or on top of your liver.
3. Now move your eyes and/or hands from side to side for about eighteen sets. Then make spiraling movements with them, making little circles that get bigger and bigger for about eighteen sets. Then reverse the direction of the spiraling and make big circles that get smaller and smaller for about twelve sets.
4. Rest for a minute. Take your mind off of the issue. Then repeat the sets of side-to-side and spiraling movements, using the same

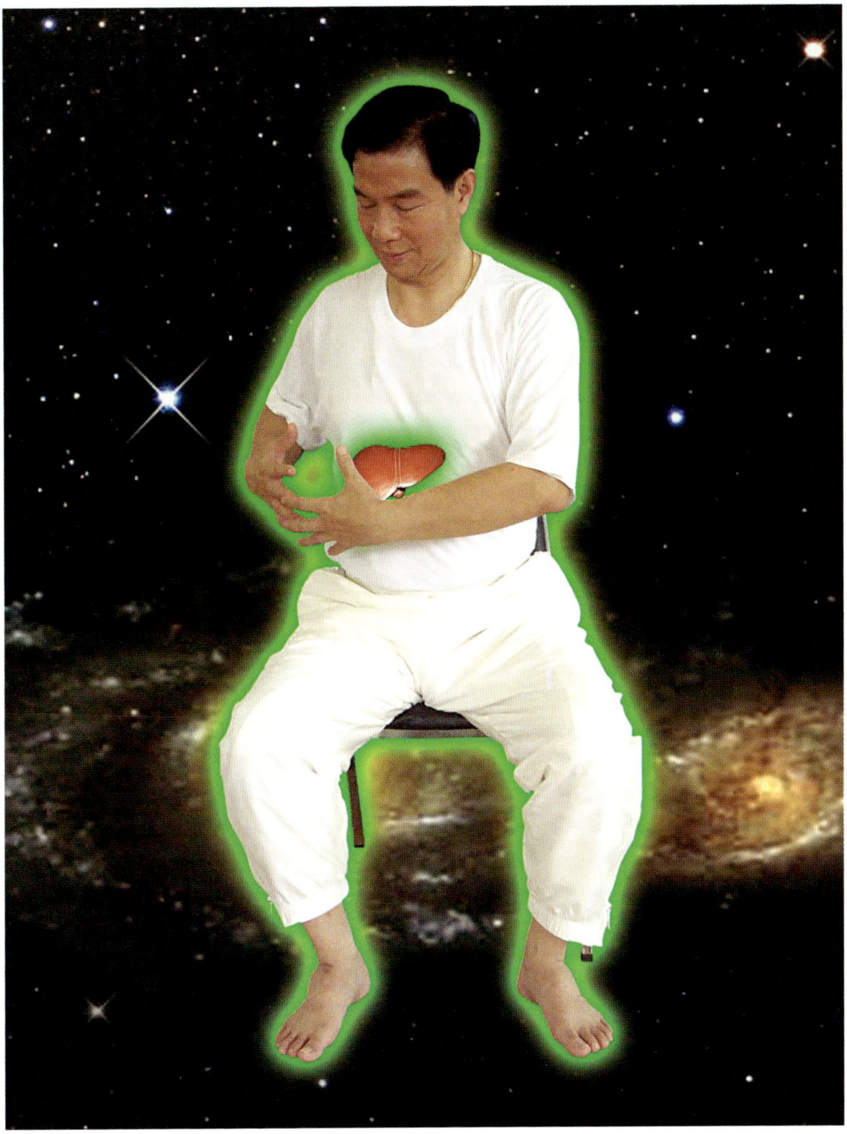

Fig. 10.7. Rebalancing and purifying negative energy in your liver.

memory to start each set, until you do not react during the processing.

5. After you complete a set of eye and/or hand movements and you think the issue may be neutralized in your liver, close your eyes and

put the starting memory back in or on top of your liver. If you do not react to the memory when you do that, then the liver does not need any more processing.

6. If you get too upset during the processing, remember to do the healing sound for the liver, *shhhhhhh*, a couple of times to calm down and cool your liver.

Dissolve the Connection between your Liver and Center of Happiness

Now return the memory to your forehead and delete, recycle, and transform in that area again for one set of the eye and/or hand movements, using the side-to-side and spiraling movements in each direction. Rest. You have completed the entire process.

STORING ACCUMULATED CHI

After you have finished practicing for the day or for the time being, it's a good idea to store the chi that you have produced. Your Lower Tan Tien can store energy. If you store the chi you cultivate every time, eventually you will have more energy stored than you need each day. When you press on your lower abdomen when it is relaxed, it will feel springy, like a full balloon, instead of squishy or empty. When you store excess chi by spiraling and packing it, you will have a reserve of energy for when life is more challenging or stressful. The process of spiraling and packing chi is slightly different for men and women.

- **Men:** Cover your navel with your right palm. Place your left palm on top of your right palm. Massage your lower abdomen with a clockwise spiraling motion, slowly making small circles that get bigger and bigger, for thirty-six rotations. Now reverse the direction and spiral inward toward your navel for twenty-four rotations.

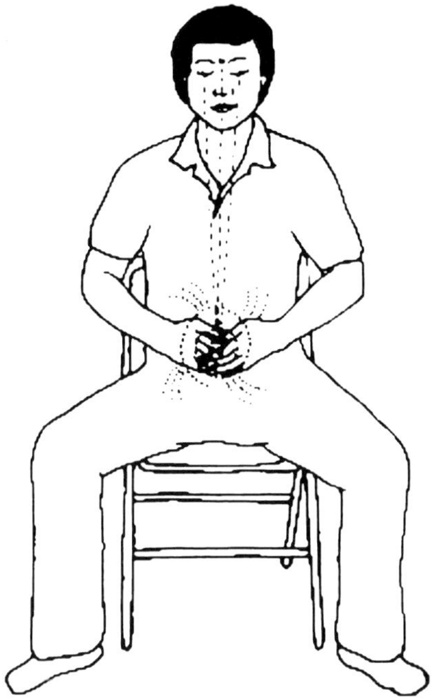

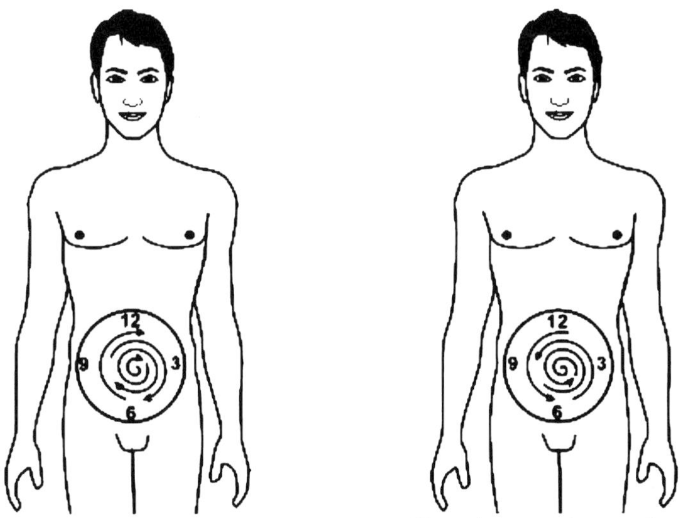

Men collect the energy by spiraling outward from the navel 36 times clockwise.

Then they spiral inward 24 times counterclockwise, ending at the navel.

Fig. 10.8. How men store chi.

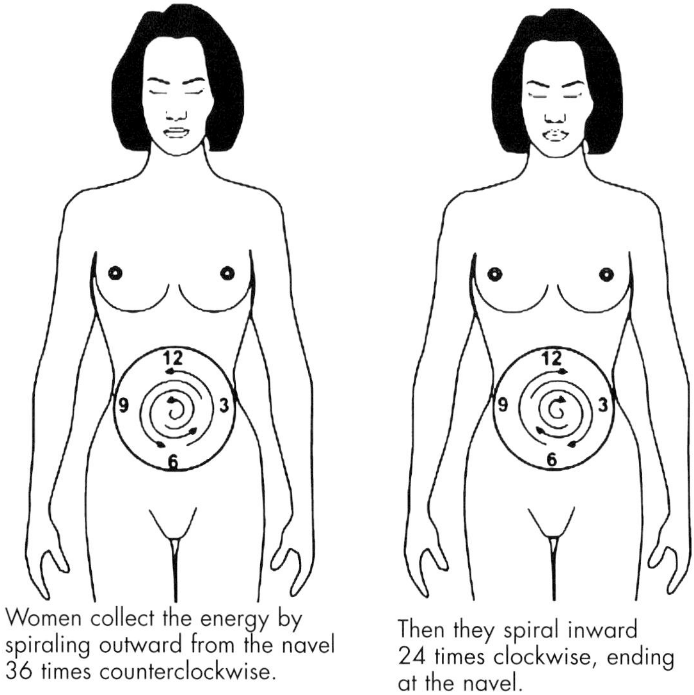

Fig. 10.9. How women collect and store energy.

- **Women:** For women, the direction of the spiraling is the opposite of what men use. Cover your navel with your left palm. Then place your right palm on top of your left palm. Massage your lower abdomen with a clockwise spiraling motion, slowly making small circles that get bigger and bigger for thirty-six rotations. Now reverse direction and spiral inward toward your navel for twenty-four rotations.

Appendix

More Recovery Resources

The practices that have been offered in this book are part of the vast system of ancient knowledge that is Taoism. All of the exercises we offer here will definitely help people effectively maintain their recovery. There are other practices in the Universal Healing Tao—too many to include here—that can provide additional benefits for those recovering from an addiction.

RECOMMENDED UNIVERSAL HEALING TAO BOOKS

Tai Chi Chi Kung is a moving practice with many physical benefits, such as stretching and strengthening the psoas muscles, twisting the spine, and stretching and strengthening the tendons. This practice also teaches people how to deal with change and to move with the flow of life. It is an energetic practice that teaches people in recovery how to live life on its terms.

Chi Self-Massage teaches people how to direct chi to a particular part of their body that needs support or healing. This practice allows people to release negative emotions, calm themselves, and rejuvenate their internal organs and nervous system. It is a quick, consequence-free, and relatively simple alternative to medicating oneself with something addictive.

Taoist Astral Healing teaches us how to connect with and draw chi from the planets and stars so that we can benefit from the different qualities of chi that originate from the heavens. The practices teach about the difference in the chi that comes from the stars and planets compared to earth energy and how to use that awareness to further balance, lighten, and strengthen one's energy body to reach one's full soul potential.

Golden Elixir Chi Kung is a practice that teaches us how to make use of the hormonal, mineral, and energetic benefits of saliva and to circulate those benefits through the whole body for optimal health. It also teaches us how to combine the energy that is produced during Taoist sexual practices with the energy from our charged saliva to create an Elixir of Immortality.

Tan Tien Chi Kung teaches people how to cultivate, condense, and store chi in their Lower Tan Tien and perineum to increase their vitality and achieve physical, mental, and spiritual balance.

Taoist Fusion meditations (***Fusion of the Five Elements, Cosmic Fusion, Fusion of the Eight Psychic Channels***) help us balance and strengthen chi by working deliberately with the elements and forces within and around us, the energy channels that bridge and regulate the channels within us, and the channels that connect their energy with the subtle energies between ourselves and other people. The result is a highly purified and powerful energy. Practicing the Fusion meditations often leads to increased awareness of the subtle signals within and around us so that we can respond more effectively to the events of our lives. The Fusion practices also teach us how to prepare our energy and guide it when we die. Learning and practicing the Fusion meditations can help people in recovery reconnect with themselves and the people around them in healthy and considerate ways.

The World Link Meditation helps us feel connected to other important people in our lives and to the universal knowledge base that is in the energy field all around us. This meditation teaches us how to fuse our observing mind, conscious mind, and mind of awareness. It teaches us how to enhance our inner peace and sense of wholeness and happiness by connecting to the energy all around us. Connecting to universal knowledge makes it easier to recognize the danger of listening to the other voices in our head that can lead us back to the path of addiction.

The Practice of Greater Kan and Li teaches us how to restore our systems to the childlike (not childish) wonder and sense of safety that we once had in childhood before life gave us experiences that led us to feel differently. The practices teach us how to invert the fire and water energies in our bodies. When combined with total darkness, the Kan and Li meditations teach us how to use that steam from the combination of fire and water to release and activate transformed sexual energy. It also stimulates the pineal gland and provides access to higher states of consciousness as a result.

Karsai Nei Tsang is a practice that involves rebalancing and strengthening the sexual energy systems in people through a combination of massage and energetic healing without touch. The practices help people release emotional and physical blockages in those areas and regulate sexual energy to treat problems such as back pain, sciatica, menopause, low libido, and hormone imbalances.

Taoist Chi Kung is famous for its treatment of sexual energy. Taoists view sexuality as powerful and healthy, not sinful or dirty. The Healing Love practices in particular give step-by-step instructions on how to make use of sexual energy for emotional, physical, mental, and spiritual benefit. There are specific practices for men, women, and couples. People in recovery from addictions can benefit not only from learning how to regulate their sexual energy so that they do not channel their addictive urges in that direction, but also so they can use those urges as raw material to create healthier energy.

All of the components of the Universal Healing Tao system work together to help people on all levels. If you want to learn more, visit MantakChia.com. On the website you can find out about the two main retreats that Master Chia offers at Tao Garden in Thailand. You can also find out about his world tour on the website. Master Chia also offers courses online. Check his pages on Facebook for current information.

Doug Hilton offers a residential treatment program for addictions at Tao Garden that incorporates the practices in this book and more. Go to www.balancerehab.solutions for more information.

Other Relevant Books by Mantak Chia

Chia, Mantak. *Energy Balance through the Tao*. Rochester, VT: Destiny Books, 2005.

———. *Iron Shirt Chi Kung*. Rochester, VT: Destiny Books, 2006.

———. *Chi Nei Tsang*. Rochester, VT: Destiny Books, 2007.

———. *The Taoist Soul Body*. Rochester, VT: Destiny Books, 2007.

———. *Healing Light of the Tao*. Rochester, VT: Destiny Books, 2008.

———. *The Inner Smile*. Rochester, VT: Destiny Books, 2008.

———. *The Six Healing Sounds*. Rochester, VT: Destiny Books, 2009.

———. *Greatest Kan and Li*. Rochester, VT: Destiny Books, 2014.

———. *The Practice of Greater Kan and Li*. Rochester, VT: Destiny Books, 2014.

———, and Christine Harkness-Giles. *Taoist Secrets of Eating for Balance: Your Personal Program for Five-Element Nutrition*. Rochester, VT: Destiny Books, 2019.

———, and Doug Hilton. *EMDR and the Universal Healing Tao: An Energy Psychology Approach to Overcoming Emotional Trauma*. Rochester, VT: Destiny Books, 2017.

———, and Lee Holden. *Simple Chi Kung*. Rochester, VT: Destiny Books, 2011.

———, and Tao Huang. *The Secret Teachings of the Tao Te Ching.* Rochester, VT: Destiny Books, 2005.

———, and Juan Li. *The Inner Structure of Tai Chi.* Rochester, VT: Destiny Books, 2005.

About the Authors

MASTER MANTAK CHIA

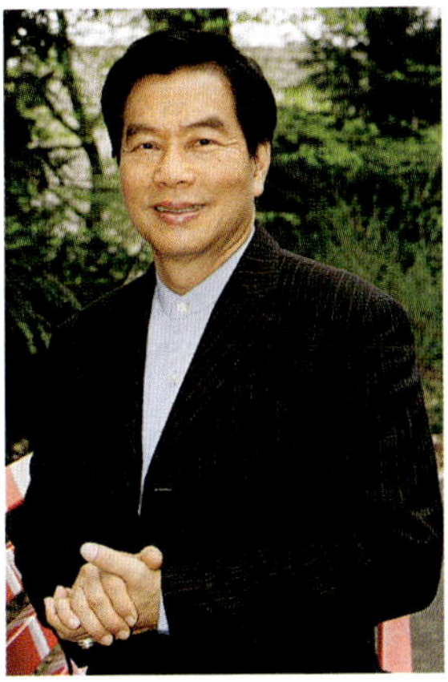

Mantak Chia has been studying the Taoist approach to life since childhood. His mastery of this ancient knowledge, enhanced by his study of other disciplines, has resulted in the development of the Universal Healing Tao system, which is now taught throughout the world.

Mantak Chia was born in Thailand to Chinese parents in 1944. When he was six years old, he learned from Buddhist monks how to sit and "still the mind." While in grammar school he learned traditional Thai boxing, and he soon went on to acquire considerable skill in aikido, yoga, and Tai Chi. His studies of the Taoist way of life began in earnest when he was a student in Hong Kong, ultimately leading to his mastery of a wide variety of esoteric disciplines, thanks to the guidance of several masters, including Master Yi Eng (I Yun), Master Meugi, Master Cheng Yao-Lun, and Master Pan Yu. To better understand the mechanisms behind healing energy, he also studied Western anatomy and medical sciences.

Master Chia has taught his system of healing and energizing practices to tens of thousands of students and trained more than three thousand instructors and practitioners throughout the world. Stemming from his teaching corps, there are established centers for Taoist study and training in many countries around the globe. Master Mantak Chia has been the only person named twice by the International Congress of Chinese Medicine and Qi Gong (Chi Kung) as Qi Gong Master of the Year (in 1990 and 2012). He was also listed as number 18 of the 100 most spiritually influential people in *The Watkins Review* in 2012.

DOUG HILTON

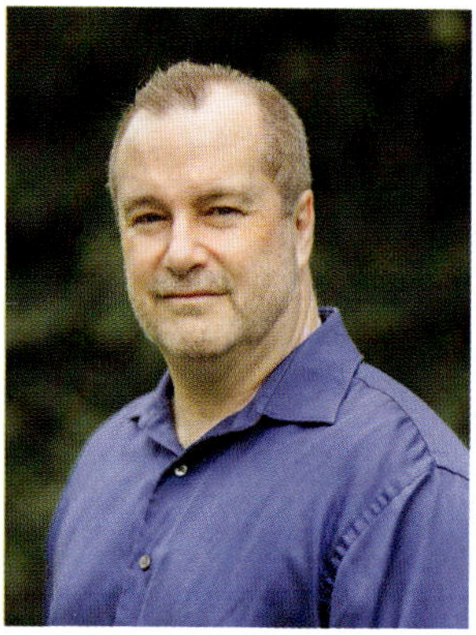

Doug Hilton holds a master's degree in counseling psychology from the University of Calgary and has worked in the counseling field for more than thirty years. Doug resides in Victoria, British Columbia, Canada, and he provides counseling services online for people of all ages all over the world, in small centers and big cities. His work experiences have provided him with specialized training and experience working with mental health concerns, marriage and family issues, trauma, and addiction. Doug has experience in many different aspects of addiction treatment, including outpatient treatment, detox (withdrawal management), day treatment, DEW (day/evening/weekend) treatment, and intensive residential treatment. He has worked extensively with gambling addiction issues for more than twenty years. He is also a Universal Healing Tao instructor and practitioner. Doug and Master Chia wrote the book *EMDR and the Universal Healing Tao: An Energy Psychology Approach to Overcoming Emotional Trauma*. Doug's websites are:

fullcirclehealing.ca and **balancerehab.solutions**

The Universal Healing Tao System and Training Center

THE UNIVERSAL HEALING TAO SYSTEM

The ultimate goal of Taoist practice is to transcend physical boundaries through the development of the soul and the spirit within the human being. That is also the guiding principle behind the Universal Healing Tao, a practical system of self-development that enables individuals to complete the harmonious evolution of their physical, mental, and spiritual bodies. Through a series of ancient Chinese meditative and internal energy exercises, the practitioner learns to increase physical energy, release tension, improve health, practice self-defense, and gain the ability to heal him- or herself and others. In the process of creating a solid foundation of health and well-being in the physical body, the practitioner also creates the basis for developing his or her spiritual potential by learning to tap into the natural energies of the sun, moon, Earth, stars, and other environmental forces.

The Universal Healing Tao practices are derived from ancient techniques rooted in the processes of nature. They have been gathered and integrated into a coherent, accessible system for well-being that works directly with the life force, or chi, that flows through the meridian system of the body.

Master Chia has spent years developing and perfecting techniques for teaching these traditional practices to students around the world through ongoing classes, workshops, private instruction, and healing sessions, as well as through books and videos and audio products. Further information can be obtained at MantakChia.com.

THE UNIVERSAL HEALING TAO TRAINING CENTER

The Tao Garden Resort and Training Center in northern Thailand is the home of Master Chia and serves as the worldwide headquarters for Universal Healing Tao activities. This integrated wellness, holistic health, and training center is situated on eighty acres surrounded by the beautiful Himalayan foothills, near the historic walled city of Chiang Mai. The serene setting includes flower and herb gardens ideal for meditation, open-air pavilions for practicing Chi Kung, and a health and fitness spa.

The center offers classes year-round, as well as summer and winter retreats. It can accommodate two hundred students, and group leasing can be arranged. For information on courses, books, products, and other resources, see below.

Universal Healing Tao Center
274 Moo 7, Luang Nua, Doi Saket, Chiang Mai, 50220 Thailand
Tel: (66)(53) 921-200
E-mail: universaltao@universal-tao.com
Website: universal-tao.com
For information on retreats and the health spa, contact:
Tao Garden Health Spa & Resort
Website: mantakchia.com/tao-garden

Index

BOOKS OF RELATED INTEREST

Chi Nei Tsang
Chi Massage for the Vital Organs
by Mantak Chia

The energies of negative emotions, stress, and tension, and the weight of past illnesses, all accumulate in the abdominal center, causing energy blockages and congestion. When this occurs, all vital functions stagnate and myriad problems arise. Practicing the self-healing techniques of Chi Nei Tsang removes this stagnation and detoxifies and rejuvenates the vital organs.

EMDR and the Universal Healing Tao
An Energy Psychology Approach to Overcoming Emotional Trauma
by Mantak Chia and Doug Hilton

Through the energy psychology practices from the 5000-year-old Taoist Chi Kung system, you can recycle negative emotional states into positive energy for your spiritual, emotional, and physical benefit. Mantak Chia and Doug Hilton provide illustrated step-by-step instructions through combining the eye movements of EMDR therapy with the energetic practices of the Universal Healing Tao.

Taoist Cosmic Healing
Chi Kung Color Healing Principles for Detoxification and Rejuvenation
by Mantak Chia

Taoist Cosmic Healing teaches the reader how to use the major acupuncture points in the hands to activate, open, and balance the chi meridians throughout the body. This practice allows the student to detoxify and rejuvenate the major organ systems and harness the astral energies of specific stars to heal others. Master Chia also presents for the first time in the West the details of Chi Kung color therapy.